Manual on Gynec Endoscopy *Techniques, Tips & Training*

68th All India Congress of Obstetrics & Gynaecology

aicog Delhi 2026

Advocate Innovate Challenge Optimise Globalise

Manual on
Gynec Endoscopy
Techniques, Tips & Training

Series Editors

Ashok Kumar
MD PhD
Director–Professor
Department of Obstetrics and Gynecology
Atal Bihari Vajpayee Institute of Medical Sciences
and Dr Ram Manohar Lohia Hospital
New Delhi, India

Madhavi M Gupta
MS
Director–Professor
Department of Obstetrics and Gynecology
Maulana Azad Medical College and Lok Nayak Hospital
New Delhi, India

K Aparna Sharma
MBBS MD
Professor
Department of Obstetrics and Gynecology
All India Institute of Medical Sciences
New Delhi, India

Editors

Sejal Naik
Ritu Vaibhav Jain
Subash Mallya
Aastha Aggrawal
Jyoti Bali
Shivani Sabharwal

JAYPEE BROTHERS MEDICAL PUBLISHERS
The Health Sciences Publisher
New Delhi | London

Message from Series Editors

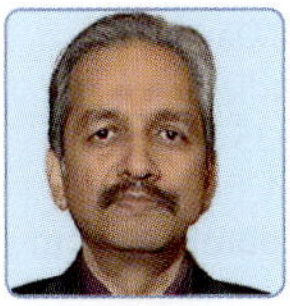

Ashok Kumar
Organizing Chairperson
AICOG-2026
New Delhi

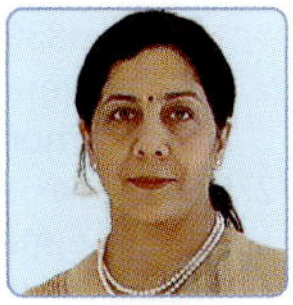

Madhavi M Gupta
Organizing Secretary
AICOG-2026
New Delhi

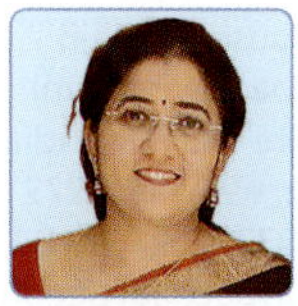

K Aparna Sharma
Organizing Secretary
AICOG-2026
New Delhi

It is after 18 long years that the 68th AICOG is being held in New Delhi. It is a pleasure to welcome you all.

The Organizing Team have poured their heart and soul into curating an academic program which one will feel a loss if missed. The scientific sessions include both national and international faculty who are stalwarts in their fields. There are 18 workshops with 8 full-day and 5 each in the pre-lunch and post-lunch time.

On this occasion, the workshop faculty, have gone that extra mile to publish the workshop manual for eight workshops. This includes all recent scientific evidence and clinical management guidelines. These manuals will serve as a go-to evidence-based resource in your day-to-day clinical practice. We look forward to receiving your valuable feedback.

We acknowledge the hard work put in by all the editors, co-editors, and the authors, who, in spite of busy schedules and time constraints, have contributed immensely.

We would also like to thank M/s Jaypee Brothers Medical Publishers (P) Ltd, New Delhi, India, for partnering with us.

We sincerely hope that you will enjoy reading these manuals, find this manual useful, and treasure it for future use in your practical work.

We take this opportunity to wish you a memorable time during your stay in New Delhi.

Warm Regards

Jaypee Brothers Medical Publishers (P) Ltd

Headquarters
EMCA House, 23/23-B
Ansari Road, Daryaganj
New Delhi 110 002, India
Landline: +91-11-23272143, +91-11-23272703
+91-11-23282021, +91-11-23245672
e-mail: jaypee@jaypeebrothers.com

Corporate Office
4838/24, Ansari Road, Daryaganj
New Delhi 110 002, India
Phone: +91-11-43574357
Fax: +91-11-43574314
e-mail: jaypee@jaypeebrothers.com

Overseas Office
JP Medical Ltd.
83, Victoria Street, London
SW1H 0HW (UK)
Phone: +44-20 3170 8910
e-mail: info@jpmedpub.com

EU GPSR Authorised Representative
Logos Europe, 9 rue Nicolas Poussin
17000, La Rochelle, France
Phone: +33 (0) 6 67 93 73 78
e-mail: contact@logoseurope.eu

Website: www.jaypeebrothers.com
Website: www.jaypeedigital.com

Inquiries for bulk sales may be solicited at: jaypee@jaypeebrothers.com

Manual on Gynec Endoscopy: Techniques, Tips & Training

First Edition: **2026**

ISBN: 978-93-7545-862-3

Printed at: Samrat Offset Pvt. Ltd.

Contributors

Aarti Chitkara Wadhawan MD DNB
Consultant
Department of Obstetrics and Gynecology
Prisma Hospital
Panipat, Haryana, India

Aastha Aggarwal MBBS MS DNB FMAS FRM MICCG FICOG
Consultant
Department of Obstetrics and Endoscopic Reconstructive-Cosmetic Urogynecology
Cloudnine Hospital
New Delhi, India

Abhinibesh Chatterjee MBBS DGO DNB FRCOG (UK) FMAS Diploma in Gynec Endoscopy (Germany)
Consultant
Department of Obstetrics and Gynecology
Manipal Hospital
Kolkata, West Bengal, India

Aditi Modi MBBS MS
Consultant
Department of Obstetrics and Gynecology
Belly and Love Women's Care
Surat, Gujarat, India

Aditi Trivedi MD
Consultant
Department of Obstetrics and Gynecology
Dr Trivedi's Total Health Care and AAKAR-IVF Centre
Surya Hospital and Well Woman Centre
Sir HN Reliance Hospital
Mumbai, Maharashtra, India

Ajay Aggarwal MBBS MD DNB
Consultant and Director
Department of Gynecology
Amayra Healthcare
Chandigarh, India

Akriti Prajapati MBBS MS
Senior Resident
Department of Obstetrics and Gynecology
Dr Kamlesh Tandon Test Tube Baby Centre
Agra, Uttar Pradesh, India

Amit Tandon MBBS MS MRCOG (1)
Gyne Laparoscopic Surgeon, Cancer Surgeon, Infertility Specialist and Robotic Surgeon
Department of Obstetrics and Gynecology
Dr Kamlesh Tandon Test Tube Baby Centre
Agra, Uttar Pradesh, India

Ankita Sharma MBBS MD
Fellow, ICOG
Department of Obstetrics and Gynecology, Endoscopy
Clio Mother and Child Institute
Ludhiana, Punjab, India

Atul Ganatra MBBS MD DGO FICOG
Consultant
Department of Obstetrics and Gynecology
Fortis and Jupiter Hospitals
Mumbai, Maharashtra
Director
Department of Obstetrics and Gynecology
Dr RJ Ganatra Nursing Home and Progeny IVF Centre
Maharashtra, India

Chintana Chandra MD
Consultant
Department of Minimally Invasive Gynecology
Endoworld Hospital
Chhatrapati Sambhajinagar
Maharashtra, India

Dinesh Kansal MBBS MD
Head and Director
Department of Obstetrics and Gynecology
BLK-Max Super Specialty Hospital
New Delhi, India

Divya TN MBBS MS
Senior Resident
Department of Minimally Invasive Gynecological Surgery
Baby Memorial Hospital
Kozhikode, Kerela, India

Freni Shah MBBS DNB MNAMS
Consultant
Department of Obstetrics and Gynecology
Fortis Hospital, Mumbai
Associate Consultant
Dr RJ Ganatra Nursing Home and Progeny IVF Centre
Mumbai, Maharashtra, India

Kalpana Choudhury MBBS MD
Senior Consultant and Endoscopic Surgeon
Department of Obstetrics and Gynecology
Health City Hospital
Guwahati, Assam, India

Kalyan B Barmade
MBBS DNB FCPS DGO DFP
Chief Director
Department of Obstetrics and Gynecology
Latur Fertility Centre Pvt Ltd, Latur
Barmade Hospital
Latur, Maharashtra, India

Kanika Jain
MBBS DGO DNB FICMCH FICOG Fellowships in Gynae Robotics and Endoscopic Surgeries
Senior Consultant, Gyne Endoscopic and Robotic Surgeon
Department of Gyne MAS sub-Specialty, Obstetrics and Gynecology
Sir Ganga Ram Hospital
New Delhi, India

Kanta M Rahul MBBS MD
Principal Consultant
Department of Anesthesia
BLK-Max Super Specialty Hospital
New Delhi, India

Kaustav Kar MBBS MD
Consultant Obstetrician, Gynecologist and Infertility Specialist
Mediland Hospital and Research Centre
Silchar, Assam, India

Maithili Kumari MBBS MD
Assistant Professor
Department of Obstetrics and Gynecology, Advanced Gynecological Endoscopic Surgery
Mahatma Gandhi Medical College and Hospital
Jaipur, Rajasthan, India

Mala Raj
MBBS DGO FICOG Dip Endoscopic Surgery Dip Reproductive Medicine (Germany)
Managing Director
Department of Obstetrics and Gynecology
Firm Hospitals
Chennai, Tamil Nadu, India

Mrinal Chatterjee
MBBS MS DNB
Fellow Reproductive Medicine
Department of Reproductive Medicine
Her Health Hospital
Bhopal, Madhya Pradesh, India

Munjal Pandya MBBS MS FICOG
Associate Professor
Department of Obstetrics and Gynecology, Endoscopy
Narendra Modi Medical College
Ahmedabad, Gujarat, India

Nikita Trehan
MBBS DNB Fellowship in Laparoscopic Surgery
Consultant Gynecological and Laparoscopic Surgeon
Sunrise Hospital
New Delhi, India

Pandit Palaskar MD DNB DFP
Director
Department of Minimally Invasive Gynecology
Endoworld Hospital
Chhatrapati Sambhajinagar
Maharashtra, India

Parul Kotadawala MBBS MD
Head
Department of Obstetrics and Gynecology, Endoscopy
VS Hospital
Ahmedabad, Gujarat, India

PG Paul MBBS DGO
Chairman and Consultant
Department of Endoscopy
Paul's Hospital
Kochi, Kerala, India

Prakash Trivedi
MBBS MD DNB DGO FCPS FICOG
Director and Head
Department of Obstetrics and Gynecology
Dr Trivedi's Total Health Care and AAKAR-IVF Centre
Mumbai, Maharashtra, India

Priya Bhave Chittawar MBBS MD
Chief Consultant and Director
Department of Obstetrics and Gynecology
Reproductive Medicine and Endoscopy Specialist, Her Health Hospital
Bhopal, Madhya Pradesh, India

R Hepshiba
MBBS DNB (Obs & Gyne) ICOG-Fellowship in Ultrasound
Consultant
Department of Obstetrics and Gynecology
Tanvir Hospital
Hyderabad, Telangana, India

Ritu Jain
MBBS MS MICOG FMAS CIMP FICOG
Director and Consultant, Professor, and Clinical Associate
Department of Obstetrics and Gynecology
Shri Mahaveer Hospital, Raipur
RIMS Medical College, Raipur
Medisure Hospital, Raipur
Chhattisgarh, India

Sejal Naik MBBS MS FMAS FRM FICOG
Director
Department of Obstetrics and Gynecology
Belly and Love Women's Care Hospital
Surat, Gujarat, India

Shivani Bedi
MBBS MD Fellowships in Gynae Robotics and Endoscopic Surgeries
Senior Resident and Gyne Endoscopic and Robotic Surgeon
Department of Gyne MAS Subspecialty, Obstetrics and Gynecology
Sir Ganga Ram Hospital
New Delhi, India

Sonia Naik MBBS MD
Principal Director
Department of Obstetrics and Gynecology, Endoscopy
Max Super Specialty Hospital
New Delhi, India

Soumil Trivedi DNB FMIGS FICOG
Co-Director and Consultant
Department of Obstetrics and Gynecology
Dr Trivedi's Total Health Care and AAKAR-IVF Center
Mumbai, Maharashtra, India

Subash Mallya
DNB DGO MNAMS Diploma in Gyn Endoscopy (Germany)
Head
Department of Minimally Invasive Gynecological Surgery
Baby Memorial Hospital
Kozhikode, Kerela, India

Supriya Mahipal MBBS MS
Associate Consultant
Department of Obstetrics and Gynecology
BLK-Max Super Specialty Hospital
New Delhi, India

Tanvir Singh MBBS MS
Consultant
Department of Obstetrics and Gynecology, Endoscopy and Urogynecology
Tanvir Hospital
Hyderabad, Telangana, India

Venus Bansal MBBS MD
Senior Consultant
Department of Obstetrics and Gynecology and Endoscopy
Clio Mother and Child Institute
Ludhiana, Punjab, India

Vijay Nahata
MBBS MD Fellow Endoscopic Surgery
Professor and Director
Department of Obstetrics and Gynecology
Advanced Gynecological Endoscopic Surgery
Mahatma Gandhi Medical College and Hospital
Jaipur, Rajasthan, India

Vivek Marwah
MBBS MD
Head
Department of Minimally Invasive Gynecology
Max Super Specialty Hospital
New Delhi, India

Yamini Kansal
MBBS MD Mch
Associate Professor
Department of Gynec Oncology
Shri Guru Ram Rai Institute of Medical and Health Sciences
Dehradun, Uttarakhand, India

Preface

From Editors Desk,

In the delicate dance of pixels and sutures, Surgery becomes an 'ART.'

In the realm of healing—where precision meets compassion—this book unfolds as a tapestry of wisdom, woven by the hands of legends in minimally invasive gynecologic surgery.

Within these pages, laparoscopy unfolds like a landscape of possibilities. With each chapter, we journey through challenges transformed into opportunities—guided by the silent strength of Anesthesia, from gentle confident Entries, the finesse of energy devices to mastering complications, each chapter whispers lessons from those who have walked the fine line between challenge and triumph. Whether you are setting up a low-cost operating room or facing the unexpected in surgery, this book offers clarity, courage, and clinical key messages.

From conquering adherent bladders to managing uterine bleeding, supporting the vault, and preventing the shadows of hemorrhage, this manual equips the surgeon with knowledge refined by experience. fertility surgery, endometriosis, burch colposuspension, and complication management—each subject is explored with depth and relevance.

In the intimate realm of hysteroscopy, innovation flows with elegance. Procedures are demystified for clarity, techniques refined to heal, and real-world insights illuminate the path for every gynecologic endoscopist with wisdom to turn obstacles into pathways. Here, the whispers of mentors become your inner voice.

Together, these sections weave a tapestry of skill and compassion, guiding you through!

The Art of Surgery is the poetry of care, written in the language of Touch.

To every graduate, colleague, and seeker of excellence—this book is your steadfast companion. Absorb the tips, embrace the tricks, and walk with the courage passed down by those who have dared and done. Learn, unlearn, and relearn—because in surgery, as in life, growth never ends.

As editors, we are honored to curate this symphony of knowledge. Within these pages lies not just instruction, but inspiration.

With gratitude to every contributor, we offer this work to you with hope that it fuels your journey in advancing women's health—with wisdom, skill, and unwavering compassion.

Elevate the touch. Transform the care. Go conquer the field, my friends!!

Warm regards,
Honored to curate this masterpiece—the Editors

Editors: **Sejal Naik, Ritu Vaibhav Jain, Subash Mallya, Aastha Aggrawal, Jyoti Bali, Shivani Sabharwal**

Contents

SECTION 1: Laparoscopy

SECTION 2: Hysteroscopy

1 SECTION

Laparoscopy

1

CHAPTER

Cost-effective and Sustainable Operation Theater Setup

Kanika Jain, Shivani Bedi

INTRODUCTION

An operation theater (OT) represents the pivotal space in any surgical facility where patient safety, precision, and efficiency converge. Escalating healthcare costs, resource constraints, and medicolegal challenges have made the creation of *sustainable, cost-effective OTs* a growing necessity worldwide.

A sustainable OT reduces environmental burden, optimizes the use of energy and resources, and supports the highest standards of surgical care within reasonable cost without compromising patient outcomes.

In India, where surgical volumes are high and resources variable, sustainability measures must balance practicality with affordability.

This is particularly relevant in obstetrics and gynecology, where the rise of Endoscopic and Robotic procedures demands an intelligent balance between technology and operational affordability.

PRINCIPLES OF COST-EFFECTIVENESS AND SUSTAINABILITY

"Cost-effectiveness" in OT design is achieved by delivering optimal patient outcomes and process efficiency while minimizing wasteful expenditure.

"Sustainability" emphasizes long-term environmental stewardship through judicious use of materials, energy, and waste management systems.

When harmonized, these principles form the backbone of a *green operating theater*—one that is efficient, economical, and environmentally responsible.

A "cost-effective and sustainable OT" integrates modular planning, reusable instruments, energy-efficient systems, and streamlined workflow **(Flowchart 1)**.

Flowchart 1: Framework for sustainable OT setup.

Planning → Infrastructure Optimization → Energy Efficiency → Equipment Utilization → Waste Management → Feedback → Audit → Continuous Improvement.

The objective is not only to save money but to extend the operational lifespan of equipment and reduce the overall carbon footprint of the surgical process.

DESIGN AND INFRASTRUCTURE OPTIMIZATION

A *modular OT design* allows flexible configuration, quick expansion, and ease of maintenance. This is the main foundation of cost effective and sustainable OTs.

Essential features include:

- Seamless, absolutely flat anti-static flooring **(Fig. 1)**
- Smooth wall panels with non-inflammable materials and laminar airflows **(Fig. 1)**
- Positive air pressure with HEPA filters maintaining at least 20 air changes per hour to ensure infection control.
- Sound insulation, Hermetic sealing, sensor operated sealed doors **(Figs. 2 and 3)**
- Functional separation of spaces, sterile and hygienic environment
- Scrub zone **(Fig. 4)**, Working CSSD **(Figs. 5 to 7)** and preoperative and postoperative recovery beds are a must.
- Positioning of endoscopic stacks **(Fig. 1)**, anesthesia workstations **(Fig. 8)**, and ceiling-mounted monitors **(Fig. 9)**, OT lights **(Fig. 10)**, Ceiling lights **(Fig. 11)**, Endoscopic equipment panels etc. to allow unhindered movements, clear sight lines **(Fig. 12)** and an Ergonomically congenial working environment for surgeons, anesthetists and staff , without trailing cables on the floor **(Table 1)**.

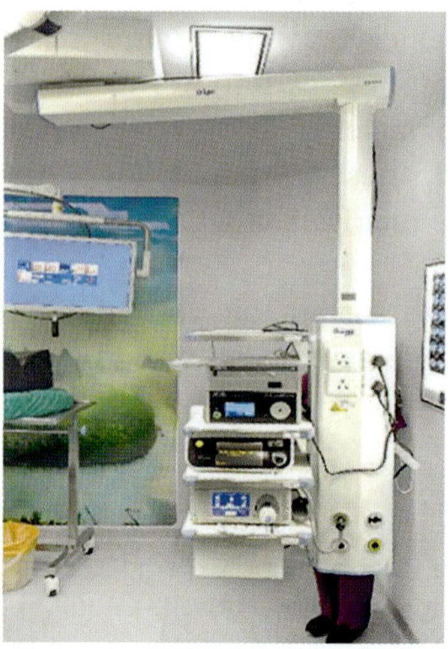

Fig. 1: Ceiling mounted monitor arm and endoscopy trolley. Also seen are seamless flooring and stainless steel wall panels.

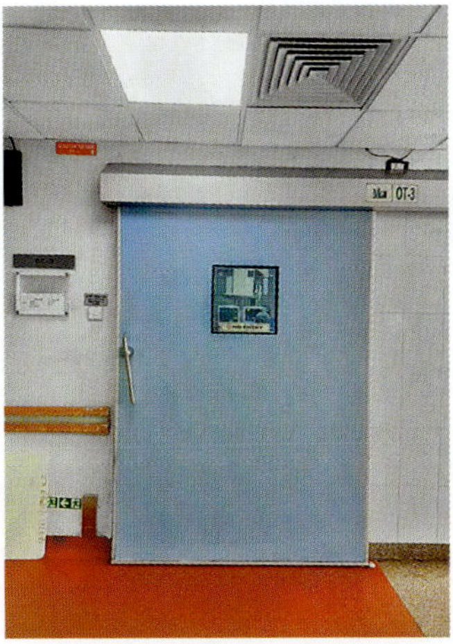

Fig. 2: Hand and foot operated sensor door of a single OT.

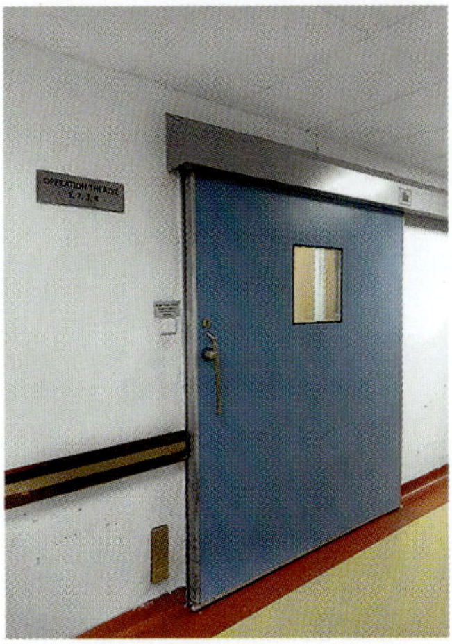

Fig. 3: Hand and foot operated sensor door of an OT complex.

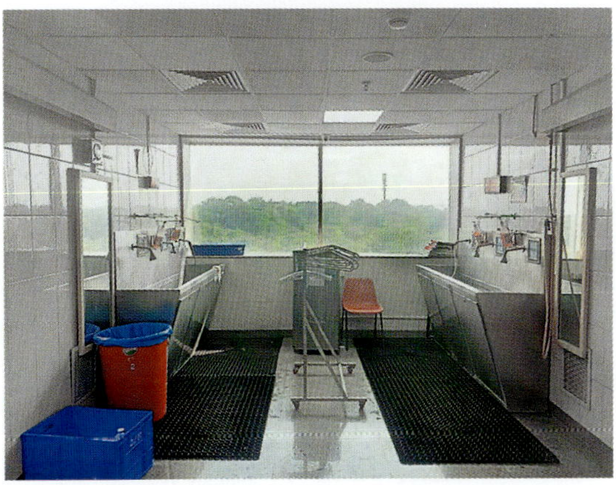

Fig. 4: Clean and well-lit Scrub Zone with sensor Taps and soap dispensers.

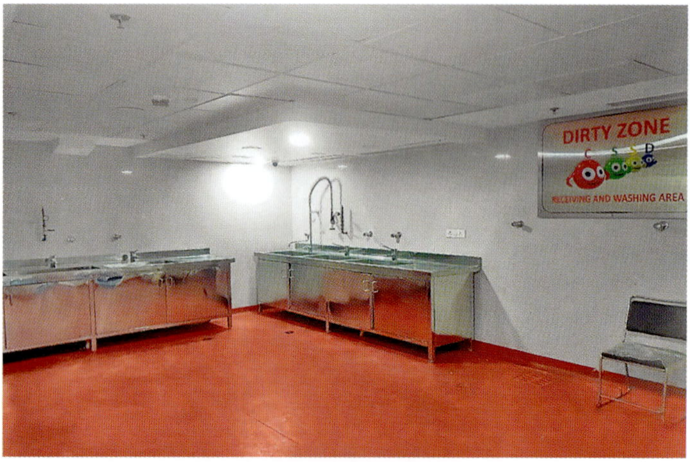

Fig. 5: Clean cleaning and washing area of CSSD.

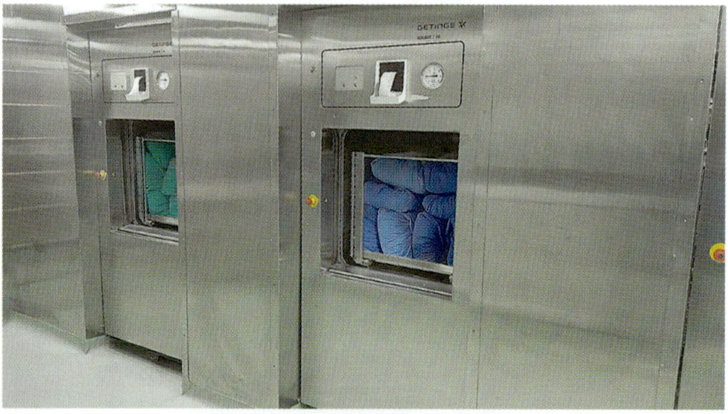

Fig. 6: CSSD autoclaving units.

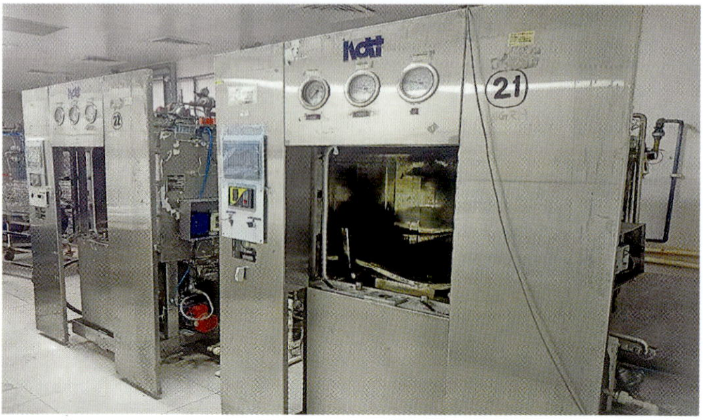

Fig. 7: CSSD autoclaving units.

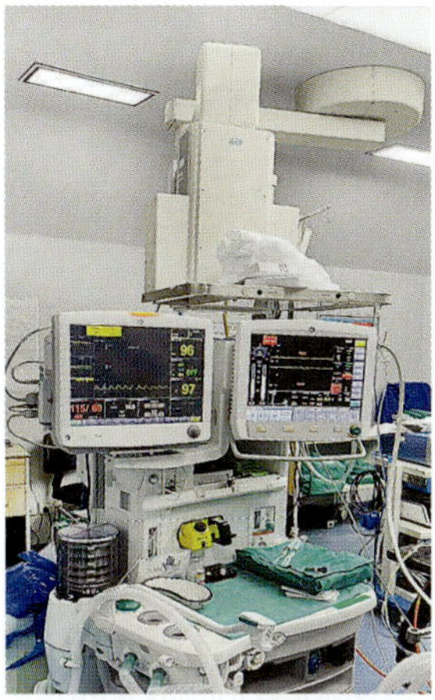

Fig. 8: Integrated ceiling mounted monitors and anesthesia workstation.

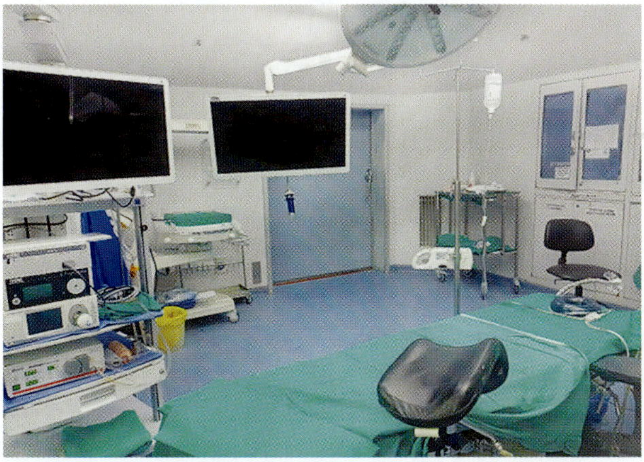

Fig. 9: Modular OT with integrated ceiling mounted monitor.

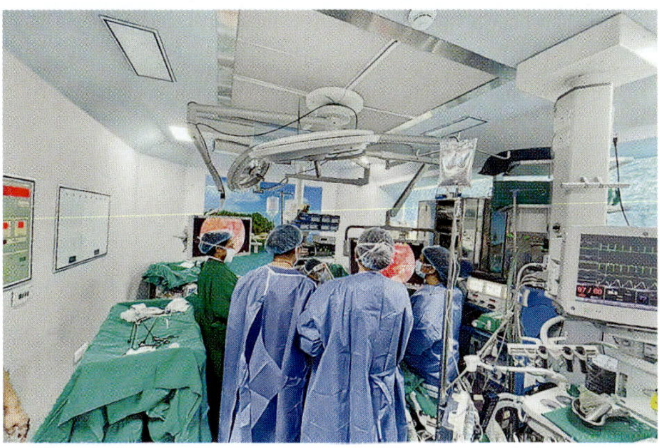

Fig. 10: Modular OT with integrated ceiling mounted monitors and OT lights maintaining ergonomics for operating surgeons.

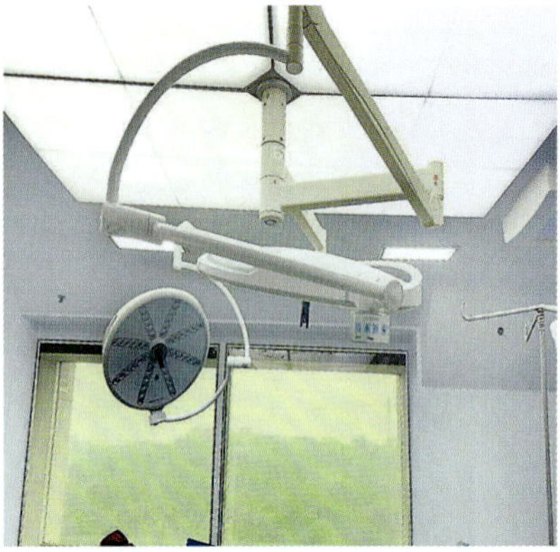

Fig. 11: Modular OT with integrated ceiling mounted OT light, ceiling lights, and large window for day light.

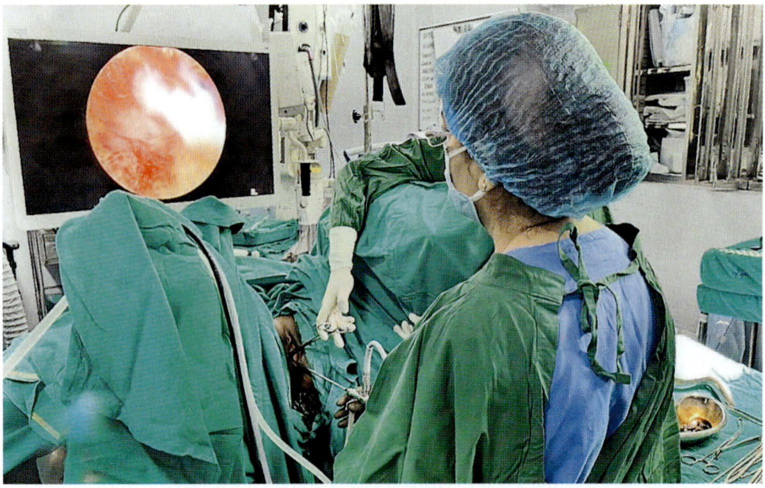

Fig. 12: Modular OT with integrated ceiling mounted monitors maintaining ergonomics for operating surgeons during hysteroscopy.

TABLE 1: Arrangement of cables and other instruments around OT table to avoid trailing and entangling of cables.

Surgeon's side	*Assistant's side*
• Wires of all energy devices • Foot pedals • Suction and irrigation tubing • Sister's instrument trolley	• Light cable • Camera cable • Insufflator tubing • Urobag

- Natural lighting **(Fig. 11)** and proper insulation to reduce dependency on artificial lighting and use of solar panels, motion sensors **(Figs. 2 and 3)**, smart lights to minimize HVAC (Heating, Ventilation and Air conditioning) load.

- Promoting Re-usable instruments, re-processing and re-cycling of single use devices, minimal use of disposable single use linens and instruments to help minimize waste and energy consumption and help reduce the carbon footprints.
- The replacement of halogen lamps with LED systems further reduces power consumption and heat production, improving both sustainability and working comfort.

ENERGY EFFICIENCY AND ENVIRONMENTAL CONTROL

Energy-efficient systems are hallmark of sustainable OTs and *green hospital ecosystem:*

- Automated lighting controls, occupancy sensors, and variable-frequency drives (VFDs) in HVAC systems can markedly reduce energy use.
- Integrating solar-assisted power backup and ensuring regular equipment calibration further improves performance and reduces costs.
- Water conservation measures, such as sensor-based taps **(Fig. 4)** and recycling of sterilization condensate, offer practical and cost-effective environmental benefits.

EQUIPMENT UTILIZATION AND MAINTENANCE IN ENDOSCOPIC OPERATION THEATERS

Endoscopic and robotic gynecological surgeries require high-end optical systems, insufflators, energy platforms, and monitors. Since these instruments represent a major cost component, careful selection and maintenance are essential.

- Equipment procurement should prioritize *multi-compatible systems* that can serve across multiple procedures, reducing duplication.
- Reusing validated sterilizable instruments such as trocars and metal cannulas, employing LED-based light sources, and shifting from consumable-based to digital recording platforms improve both sustainability and cost control.
- Standardized instrument trays also prevent the sterilization of unused tools, saving both time and energy.
- Preventive maintenance schedules and biomedical engineer involvement are critical to prolong equipment lifespan.

Although sustainable practices can involve higher initial expenses, they tend to yield strong long-term financial returns.

WORKFLOW EFFICIENCY AND MANPOWER UTILIZATION

An efficient OT is not just about physical design—it is about how teams function within that space. A well-trained multidisciplinary team, familiar with both endoscopic and open techniques, ensures flexibility and responsiveness.

- Electronic scheduling systems, real-time dashboards, and task-based role division can optimize manpower use and minimize delays for cost effective OT functionality
- Cross-training staff for both open and laparoscopic procedures helps maintain continuity during emergencies.
- Continuous audits and team debriefings ensure accountability and continuous improvement.

WASTE REDUCTION AND INFECTION CONTROL

Sustainability in OT operations extends to waste management.

- *Segregation at source, reprocessing of metallic instruments, and use of biodegradable materials* such as drapes and gloves form the foundation of eco-friendly surgical practice.
- Closed suction systems and scavenging of anesthetic gases minimize contamination risks.
- The reduction of packaging materials, proper labelling, and limited use of single-use plastics significantly lower biomedical waste volumes.
- Infection prevention protocols—like standard cleaning between cases and daily terminal cleaning—must be strictly followed to maintain sterility and patient safety.

COST OPTIMIZATION STRATEGIES

A comprehensive cost-optimization framework should address lighting, equipment, consumables, and utilities **(Table 2)**.

Integration of the Central Sterile Supply Department (CSSD) enhances sterilization efficiency, while cycle optimization reduces energy and water consumption.

PLANNING AND ARCHITECTURAL CONSIDERATIONS

The *planning phase* should clarify surgical volume, case mix, and emergency capacity. The theater should be located near ICU, wards, CSSD, and imaging

TABLE 2: Cost optimization approaches.

Domain	*Strategy*
Lighting and Power	LED systems, motion sensors, efficient HVAC with VFD
Equipment	Preventive maintenance, resource sharing across units
Consumables	Reusable drapes/instruments, rational inventory rotation
Sterilization	CSSD integration, autoclave cycle optimization
Water Use	Sensor taps, condensate water recycling

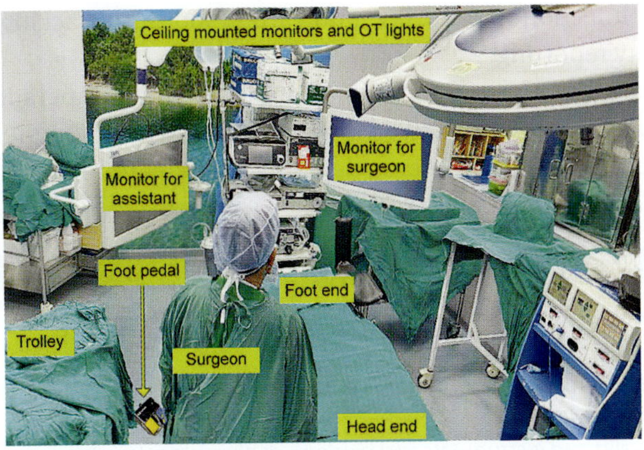

Fig. 13: Modular OT: Architectural considerations

for seamless flow. Proper zoning—protective, clean, aseptic, and disposal zones—prevents cross-contamination.

Architectural considerations include adequate room size (≥7 × 7 m; 3.5 m height), smooth seamless finishes, sliding doors, and ergonomic placement of equipment **(Fig. 13)**.

Electrical and medical gas systems must comply with international safety standards, supported by dedicated circuits and UPS backup.

HVAC design must maintain temperature (18–24°C), positive pressure gradients, and sufficient air changes per hour. Laminar flow ceilings or HEPA filtration are essential in endoscopic and high-risk surgeries.

COMPLIANCE, COMMISSIONING, AND ACCREDITATION

Compliance with standards such as NABH and NHSRC (India) ensures that OTs meet stringent safety, quality, and infection-control benchmarks.

Each OT must undergo commissioning of HVAC, medical gas systems, and electrical isolation checks before becoming operational.

Documentation of test results, cleaning protocols, and maintenance records is essential for audit and accreditation readiness.

Lifecycle budgeting that includes preventive maintenance and upgrade costs helps avoid expensive retrofits later.

TECHNOLOGY INTEGRATION AND FUTURE-READINESS

Modern OTs are increasingly *digitally integrated*. Real-time monitoring of vital parameters, OR management software, and connectivity with hospital information systems (HIS) streamline operations. Integration of imaging and data within hybrid OTs enables precise, minimally invasive procedures.

Future OT systems are expected to incorporate artificial intelligence for scheduling and predictive maintenance, Internet of Things (IoT) sensors for energy and infection monitoring, and carbon footprint tracking to support sustainability reporting.

Designing the infrastructure to accommodate future upgrades—such as robotics (Bigger OTs) or advanced imaging—is critical for long-term value.

The success of these systems depends not only on design but also on *training and adaptation* among healthcare workers.

KEY POINTS

- A sustainable OT ensures patient safety, operational efficiency, and long-term cost savings.
- Energy-efficient lighting, modular infrastructure, and preventive maintenance are crucial.
- Reuse of validated instruments and biodegradable materials reduces environmental impact.
- Cross-trained staff and workflow audits sustain high performance.
- Integration of IT systems and environmental monitoring supports continuous improvement.
- Gynecological endoscopic OTs can balance advanced technology with eco-efficiency through smart procurement and shared resources.

SUGGESTED READING

1. BioMed Central. Digital and Smart Operating Theatres: Future Trends. 2023.
2. BioMed Central. Optimizing Operating Room Utilization through Scheduling Systems. 2022.
3. ETKHO Hospital Engineering. Energy and Airflow in Surgical Environments. Barcelona: ETKHO Hospital Engineering; 2020.
4. ETKHO Hospital Engineering. Hybrid Operating Theatre Concepts. Barcelona: ETKHO Hospital Engineering; 2021.
5. ETKHO Hospital Engineering. Operating Theatre Design and Standards. Barcelona: ETKHO Hospital Engineering; 2021.
6. Gupta N. Designing Energy Efficient Operating Theatres in India. Indian J Surg. 2019;81(5):521-8.
7. Healthcare Without Harm. Green Operating Theatres: Strategies for Sustainable Surgery. 2022.
8. IJMRHS. Modular OT Construction in Resource Limited Settings. 2020.
9. Lippincott Journals. Infection Control in Operation Theatres. 2021.
10. NABH. Accreditation Standards for Hospitals, 6th edition. New Delhi: NABH; 2022.
11. National Health Systems Resource Centre (NHSRC). Operational Guidelines for Operation Theatre Complex. New Delhi: NHSRC; 2021.
12. NHS England. Delivering a Net Zero National Health Service. London: NHS; 2020.
13. NHSRC India. Operational Guidelines for Operation Theatre Complex. New Delhi: NHSRC; 2021.
14. Sherman JD. Environmental Footprint of Surgical Practices. Anesth Analg. 2021;132(1):160-8.

15. Sherman JD. Life Cycle Assessment and Cost Analysis of Surgical Instrument Reuse. JAMA Surg. 2021;156(6):580-8.
16. Vanderbilt University Medical Center. Surgical Suite Design Guidelines. Nashville: Vanderbilt University Medical Center; 2020.
17. WHO. Safe Surgery Saves Lives: Infection Prevention in Surgical Care. Geneva: WHO; 2020.
18. World Health Organization. Sustainable Health Care Facilities: A Global Guide. Geneva: WHO; 2020.
19. Yadav RK. Modular Operating Theatres: A Practical Approach. Indian J Med Res Health Sci. 2020;12(3):71-4.
20. Zenodo.org. Guidelines for Hospital Operating Theatre Planning. Switzerland: European Organization for Nuclear Research; 2022.

2

CHAPTER

Energy Sources in Endoscopic Surgery

Atul Ganatra, Freni Shah

INTRODUCTION

The use of electrosurgery dates back to the 1800s with Becquerel being the pioneer of electrocautery techniques.

The earliest technique involved the usage of direct current being passed through a wire which was later replaced by the usage of alternating current of high frequency, i.e., 100 KHz. This modification prevented stimulation of nerves and muscles.

This high-frequency alternate current led to higher tissue temperatures. D'Arsonval proved this much later and his student Rivere, thus was the first to utilize electro-surgery for treatment of hand ulcer in 1900.

In 1926, Cushing used the electrosurgical generator then created by Bovie for his neurosurgical procedures. Bovie's generator advanced the adoption of electrosurgery and marked the beginning of its contemporary period.

PRINCIPLES OF ELECTROSURGERY

Electrosurgery is defined as conversion of high-frequency electric current to thermal energy. This results in tissue effects like vaporization, desiccation and coagulation.

Current (I) is flow of electrons during a period of time, like water flowing down a river. Current flows from negative to positive on the surface of a conductor. Current is measured in amperes (A) or Amps **(Fig. 1)**.

Voltage (V) is the difference in electrical potential between 2 points in a circuit.

Pushing current through the resistance and is measured in volts (V) **(Fig. 1)**.

Resistance is obstacle to the flow of current, measured in ohms.

Resistors are used to control voltage and current levels **(Fig. 1)**.

A very high resistance allows a small amount of current to flow. A very low resistance allows a large amount of current to flow. Resistance is measured in Ω ohms.

When electric current flows in one direction it is "direct". When electric current changes direction regularly, it is "alternating". Direct current is used in electrocautery whereas indirect current is used in electrosurgery.

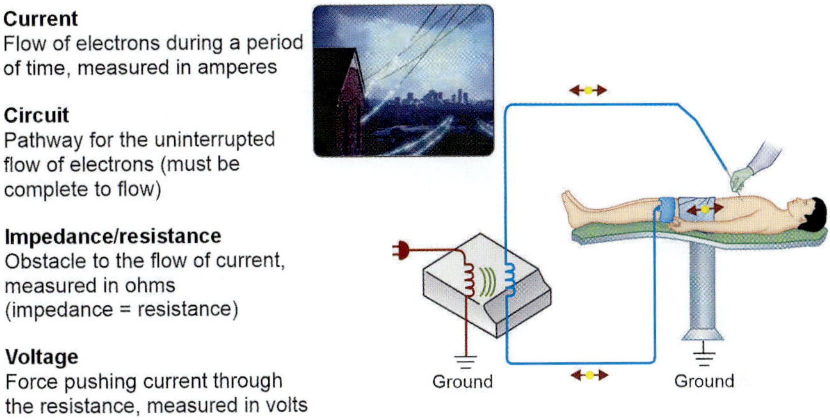

Fig. 1: Properties of electricity.

According to Ohm's law, current in amperes (Amp) is equal to the voltage in volts divided by the resistance in ohms

$$\text{Current (I)} = \text{Voltage (V)}/\text{Resistance (R)}$$

Hence in order to increase the current, we have to increase the voltage or reduce the resistance. Power is the amount of energy produced (or consumed) per unit time and is measured in watts.

$$\text{Power (P)} = \text{Voltage (V)} \times \text{Current (I) or } P = V^2/R$$

An electrosurgical unit (ESU) converts household electricity frequency (50–60 Hz) to high frequency 500,000–3,000,000 Hz thus preventing stimulation of nerves and muscles. This causes the cellular ions in the target tissue to oscillate and generate heat. This heat produces various desirable tissue effects.

A generator, two electrodes and the patient form an electro-surgical unit.

As shown in **(Figure 2A)** a monopolar circuit consists of an active electrode near the target tissue and a dispersive electrode which is attached remotely on the patient to complete the circuit and dissipate the current safely. However, in a bipolar circuit **(Figure 2B)** the electric current is confined to the tissues between the two electrodes that are near to the target tissue.

THERMAL EFFECTS

The tissue response generated by electrosurgery depends on the temperature achieved at the tissue level. Desiccation and coagulation: These effects occur when the tissue temperature gradually rises between 69 and 95°C. Sudden loss of water from the cell causes desiccation whereas denaturation of proteins causes coagulation. A wider electrode with low-density current using any of the three basic waveforms can cause these effects.

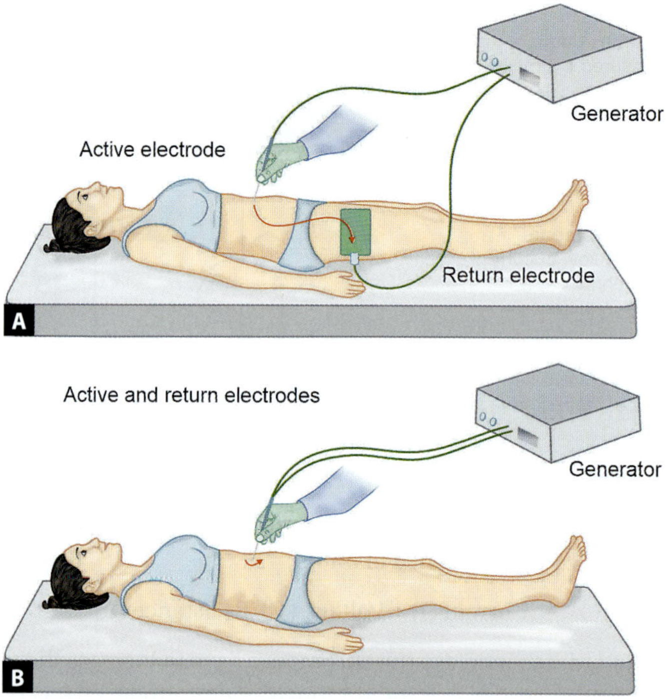

Figs. 2A and B: (A) Monopolar electrode; and (B) Bipolar electrode Vaporization: This effect occurs when the tissue temperature rapidly rises from normal to 100°C causing an explosion of cells. This effect is used for tissue cutting. With pure cut (continuous waveform with no tissue contact) setting there is minimal lateral thermal damage however when using blend or coag (intermittent waveform) for cutting the power needs to be increased to achieve the desired effect. This increase in voltage can lead to more thermal damage. Fulguration: In this the high voltage arcing between the electrode and the tissue creates a high temperature of 200°C or more causing carbonization of tissue. The electrode uses coag waveform and is not in contact with the tissue. A low duty cycle creates minimal heat in deeper layers, thus, thin carbonization layer. This is because the current diminishes rapidly. For controlling blood oozing from surfaces, fulguration is very effective. The tissue effects are not only dependent on the temperature generated but also on the following variables.

Generator mode: Every generator has three fundamental current waveforms being used in electrosurgery, i.e., cut, blend and coagulation depending on the wattage, voltage and duty cycle of the current as shown in **Figure 3**.

When hemostasis is required with cutting, this waveform is used as it can produce a combination of tissue cutting with desiccation and coagulation. Some generators have blend 1, 2 and 3 with duty cycle at 50%, 40% and 25% respectively **(Fig. 3 and Table 1)**. The higher its duty cycle the more cutting and less coagulation it produces and vice versa. As every waveform described above can produce both cutting and coagulation depending on the duty cycle, size of the electrode and contact with the tissue, the terms cut and coag modes are misleading.

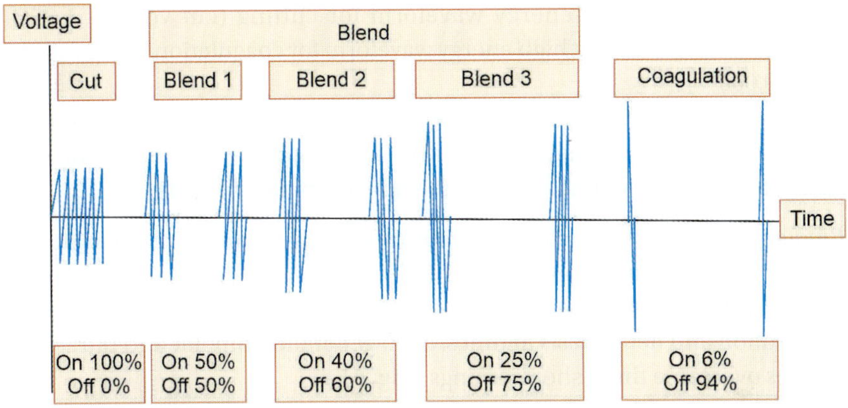

Fig. 3: Basic current waveforms with their voltage and duty cycle.

TABLE 1: Basic current waveforms with their voltage and duty cycle.

Cut mode	Continuous waveform	High current	Low voltage	100% duty cycle	Yellow coded
Coag mode	Interrupted waveform	Low current	High voltage	6% duty cycle	Blue coded
Blend mode	Modulated waveform	Variable current	Variable voltage	Variable duty cycle	Blue coded

Power setting: Power is directly proportional to the amount of voltage used.

Hence, high power means high voltage and consequently high chance of complications. Therefore, it is advisable to use the minimum possible power.

Effective cutting requires 50–80 W in the cut mode and effective coagulation requires 30–50 W in the coag mode.

Time of contact: While too short a contact time results in insufficient tissue effects, longer contact between the active electrode and tissue can lead to wider and deeper tissue effects as well as unintentional thermal injuries. The optimal contact time will minimize complications due to thermal injury.

Shape of the active electrode: An electrode used for cutting should be pointed or narrow to concentrate the density of current on the tissue while a broader electrode will cause coagulation of tissues. The electrode used in fulguration is usually spherical.

Tissue resistance: High resistance tissues (fat, fibrosed tissue) require more power to achieve the desired effect as compared to low resistance tissues with (skin, muscle).

■ VARIOUS TYPES OF ELECTROSURGICAL INSTRUMENTS

Monopolar instruments: They have been in use for a long time for cutting, coagulating, hemostasis and fulguration. These instruments make use of continuous low energy waveform for cutting (cut voltage 1,350–4,000 V) and intermittent high energy waveform for coagulation (coag voltage 3,000–9,000 V).

The maximum temperature attained after activation of instruments is >100°C. The amount of thermal spread with monopolar instruments can vary from 3.5 to 20 mm depending upon the time of contact **(Fig. 4)**.

Bipolar instruments: Bipolar instruments are safer than monopolar due to the use of less voltage power (300–1,200 V). However, coaptation of tissues was not always perfect with these instruments which resulted in incomplete coagulation and hemostasis at times. New-generation bipolar and ultrasonic devices overcame these shortcomings **(Fig. 4)**.

Advanced bipolar instruments: These instruments were developed to provide the advantage of better tissue coaptation by utilizing tissue feedback mechanism and less amount of energy. They are built in such a way that they can coagulate and seal tissues up to 7 mm in diameter and additionally transect the tissue at the same time. The use of lesser amount of energy and a pulsed manner of energy delivery causes lesser thermal spread and smoke production.

The vessel sealing devices (Ligasure™) (Valleylab Inc., Boulder, CO, USA) (LS) vessel sealing instrument **(Fig. 5)** uses a high-current (4A), low-voltage (180 V).

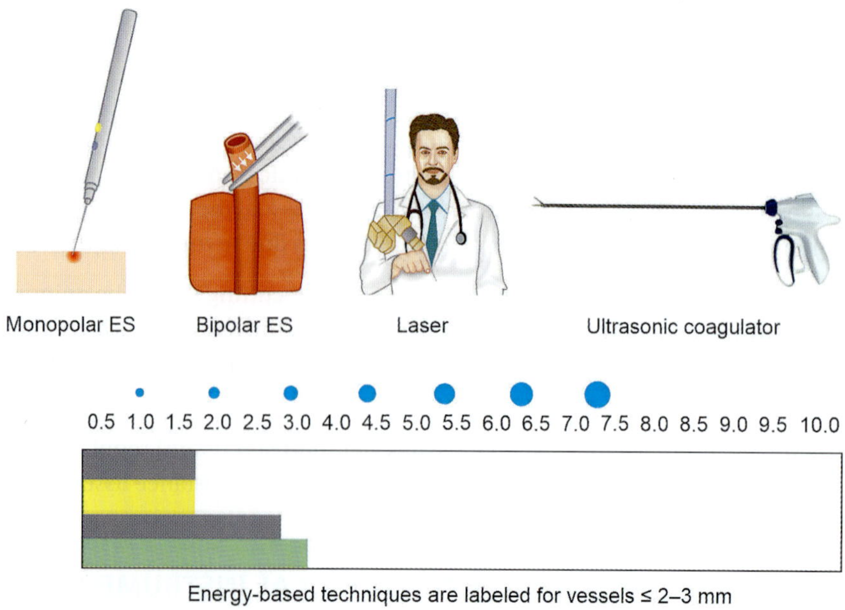

Fig. 4: Energy-based thermal devices.

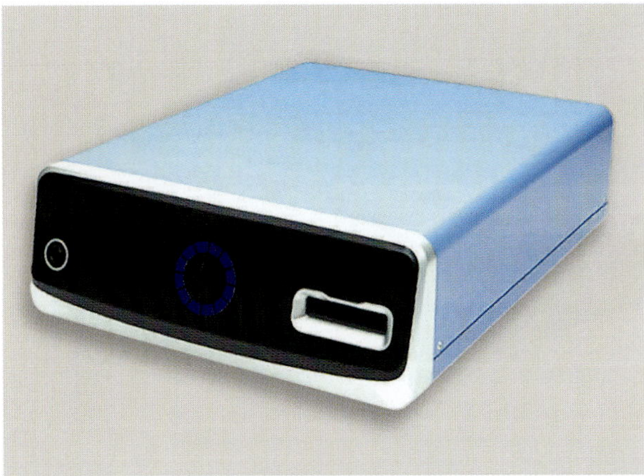

Fig. 5: Ligasure generator.

The system works by fusing the collagen in the vessel wall to create a permanent seal. The seal thus formed can withstand pressure greater than three times normal systolic pressure. It is an efficient vessel sealing device with minimal thermal spread.

ENSEAL™ (Ethicon Endo-surgery, US, LLC) this tissue-sealing and hemostasis system is a bipolar instrument combination of a high-compression jaw with a tissue dynamic energy delivery mechanism. It is designed in such a way that the amount of energy delivered at the tip (which contain the nanopolar thermostats) of the instrument changes according to the tissue impedance. Additionally, the instrument is fitted with a blade which can cut the sealed tissue.

Harmonic ACE™ (Ethicon Endo-Surgery, Cincinnati, OH, USA) **(Fig. 6)** is an ultrasonic device that converts electrical energy to vibrations by oscillating the blades of the device at a frequency of 55,000 cycles per second thus denaturing the tissue proteins and causing coagulation. The instrument consists of the transducer, hand grip, long shaft and blades. There is an inactive blade which helps in grasping the tissues and also prevents the vibrational energy from spreading further and an active blade that vibrates and denatures protein in the tissue. There are five power level settings that can produce different tissue effects. Low power setting is used for coagulation while high power setting is used for cutting.

Thunderbeat™ (Olympus Medical Systems Corp., Tokyo, Japan) (TB) **(Fig. 7)** is the first device to integrate both ultrasonically generated frictional heat energy and advanced bipolar energy in one instrument. Thus, single instrument performs both cutting and sealing using ultrasonic and bipolar energy respectively for the two tissue effects. The generator has level 1 for cutting and sealing while level 3 for sealing mode. It can seal and cut vessels up to 7 mm diameter.

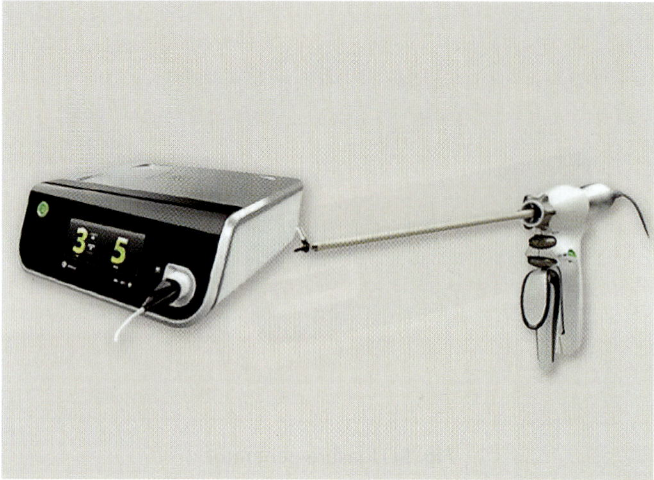

Fig. 6: Harmonic generator with curved tip shears.

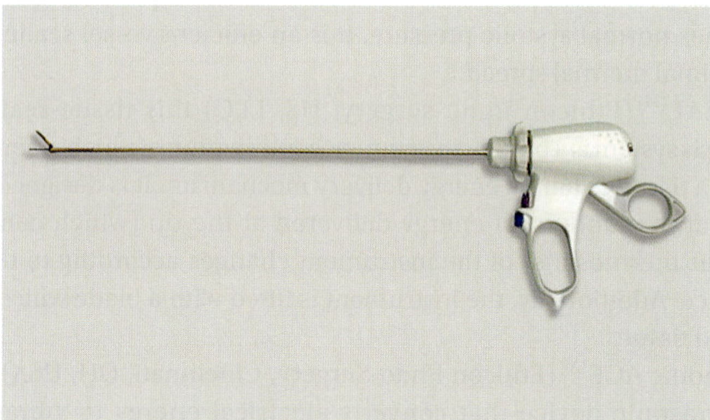

Fig. 7: Thunderbeat.

Thus, advanced bipolar instruments are not only safe but also cost-effective.

ELECTROSURGICAL HAZARDS

Like any other new technology electrosurgery also has a set of hazards associated with its use and all surgeons must be aware of them and try their best to prevent them. Accidental burns are seen to occur in 3–4 per 1,000 procedures.

Residual heat: The active electrode becomes hot after being used and therefore surgeons should avoid touching other organs with the instrument before they cool down. The amount of heat generated by ultrasonic devices is maximum as compared to other devices.

Thermal spread: This is the most common form of electrosurgical burn. It is more common with the use of monopolar. It can be avoided by keeping the power and contact time minimum.

Direct thermal extension (pedicle effect): When current is applied to a narrow structure of tissue it causes unintentional burns at the area. To avoid this usage of minimal power for short duration is recommended.

Burns at the dispersive electrode site: The dispersive electrode is kept close to the field of surgery but away from areas of high impedance like bony prominences, scar tissue, hairy and contoured body parts. When the electrode is not in proper contact with the body surface then burns happen at the application site by the end of surgical procedure. Nowadays generators have technology which detects poor contact or high impedance and gives alarm signals thus preventing complications.

Insulation failure: Laparoscopy instruments can be either single use or reusable. While reusing instruments it is important to check integrity of the instrument. Any defect in the instrument can cause leakage of current and thus injury to the part of organ which it comes in contact with during the surgery **(Fig. 8A)**. Insulation failure accidents are more commonly seen in robotic instruments. Nowadays, active electrode monitoring (AEM) system can be attached to the generator to return stary current to the AEM monitor.

Capacitive coupling: This happens when the current is induced in a conductor around an insulated activated electrode **(Fig. 8B)**. This phenomenon is common with hybrid trocars with plastic anchors as they prevent dissipation of current along the abdominal wall hence their use was abandoned. The AEM technology used in modern day generators can minimize these hazards. This hazard can be prevented by keeping safe distance between two conductors, usage of thicker insulation, use of low power setting and by decreasing the time of activation of electrode.

Direct coupling: When an active electrode comes in contact with an inactive metal instrument then it can injure any tissue that the instrument touches **(Fig. 8C)**. The surgeon needs to be vigilant where the tip of the active electrode is inside the body cavity while activating it.

Antenna coupling: In this electromagnetic energy from one cord gets captured by another nearby inactive cord (ECG wires, EEG wires, camera cord) causing burns to the patient. Hence, the laparoscopy tower must be separated from the generator to avoid this coupling.

Glove burns: These can be caused by dielectric breakdown, capacitive coupling and direct current conduction. To prevent these burns the surgeon must use minimum effective power, avoid prolonged activation of electrodes and wear double gloves or change gloves in between the surgery.

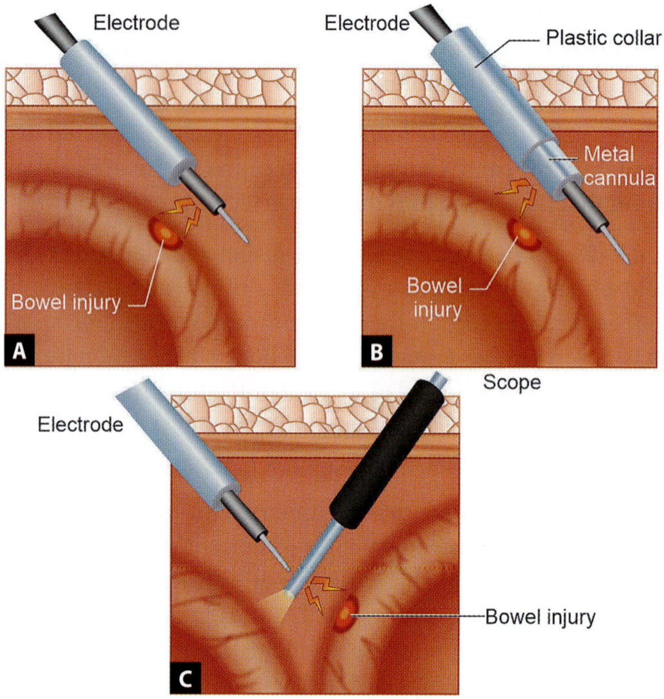

Figs. 8A to C: (A) Insulation failure; (B) Capacitive coupling; (C) Direct coupling.

Exposure to surgical smoke: Surgical smoke as a by-product of electrosurgery is made of 95% water vapor and 5% other materials. It contains toxic and mutagenic substances. Smoke particles of less than 5 microns can cause bronchiolitis, emphysema and pulmonary fibrosis when inhaled for a long time. Therefore, it is necessary for surgeons and theatre staff to wear appropriate personal protection equipment (PPE) and use closed circuit smoke evacuation devices in Operation Theater. The amount of smoke produced by bipolar and ultrasonic instruments is less as compared to monopolar instrument.

Surgical explosions: The incidence of surgical explosions has reduced nowadays with the use of pure carbon dioxide gas for creating pneumoperitoneum.

However, it is advisable to do bowel preparation before laparoscopy surgery as they can accumulate flammable gases such as hydrogen and methane which can get released during accidental perforation or intentional resection. Chapter 4: The Use of Electrosurgery in Laparoscopy Interference with electromagnetic devices: Electrosurgical instruments have the tendency to interfere with electromagnetic devices like pacemaker, defibrillators or neurostimulators and cause cardiac arrhythmias and asystole.

Hence it is important to have a multidisciplinary approach in such patients with re-programming of devices if required before or during surgery. Monopolar instruments have shown to cause more interference than bipolar or ultrasonic devices. While using monopolar devices it is advisable to use short bursts of low voltage, place dispersive electrode and avoid hovering of electrosurgical instrument over the implant device. The electrosurgical instruments have also shown to cause interference with electrocardiography (ECG) machine and video imaging systems. The best way to avoid this is to maintain adequate distance between the two electromagnetic devices.

CONCLUSION

Newer technological advances have made use of electrosurgery safer, cost-effective and surgeon friendly. A sound and correct knowledge of the basics of electrosurgery and its safe use along with proper training of the surgeon, is very essential to avoid any kind of compromise on patient safety.

SUGGESTED READING

1. El-Sayed M, Mohamed S, Saridogan E. Safe use of electrosurgery in gynaecological laparoscopic surgery. Obstet Gynaecol. 2020;22(1):9-20.
2. Espada M, Munoz R, Noble BN, Magrina JF. Insulation failure in robotic and laparoscopic instrumentation: a prospective evaluation. Am J Obstet Gynecol. 2011;205(2):121.e1-5.
3. Law KSK, Abbott JA, Lyons SD. Energy Sources for Gynecologic laparoscopic surgery: A review of the literature. Obstet Gynecol Surv. 2014;69(12):763-76.
4. Massarweh NN, Cosgriff N, Slakey DP. Electrosurgery: History, Principles, and Current and Future Uses. J Am Coll Surg. 2006;202(3):520-30.
5. Meyer JP, Crew J. The risks of diathermy in the urological patient with a pacemaker or an automatic internal cardiac defibrillator. BJU Int. 2008;101(5):528-9.
6. Munro MG. Economics and energy sources. J Minim Invasive Gynecol. 2013;20(3):319-27.
7. Sutton PA, Awad S, Perkins AC, Lobo DN. Comparison of lateral thermal spread using monopolar and bipolar diathermy, the Harmonic Scalpel™ and the Ligasure. Br J Surg. 2010;97(3):428-33.
8. The American Society of Anesthesiologists Committee on Standards and Practice Parameters. Practice advisory for the perioperative management of patients with cardiac implantable electronic devices: pacemakers and implantable cardioverter-defibrillators: an updated report by the American Society of Anesthesiologists task force on perioperative management of patients with cardiac implantable electronic devices. Anesthesiology. 2011;114(2):247-61.
9. Vilos G, Latendresse K, Gan BS. Electrophysical properties of electrosurgery and capacitive induced current. Am J Surg. 2001;182(3):222-5.
10. Wang K, Advincula AP. "Current thoughts" in electrosurgery. Int J Gynaecol Obstet. 2007;97(3):245-50.

3 CHAPTER

Anesthesia: Partner in Success, Silent in Glory

Kanta M Rahul

INTRODUCTION

Over a century ago, laparoscopy was first introduced as a therapeutic alternative to laparotomy. Since then, the field of laparoscopy has evolved and grown tremendously. Improved surgical cosmesis, reduced post-operative pain, faster return to work, and lower surgical complications makes it preferrable over open surgeries.

Anesthesia plays a pivotal role in ensuring the success of these surgeries. Though often unnoticed when outcomes are excellent, the anesthetist's vigilance underpins patient safety, physiological stability and optimal operating conditions. In this chapter we will be discussing an academic overview of perioperative anesthetic care, relevant physiology, intraoperative management and postoperative considerations for gynecological laparoscopic procedures.

LAPAROSCOPIC GYNECOLOGICAL SURGERY: BRIEF OVERVIEW

The most common indications for laparoscopy in gynecological procedures include hysterectomy, oophorectomy, myomectomy and diagnostic procedures. Laparoscopy , in principal requires CO_2 pneumoperitoneum and what makes it different for gynecological procedures is that they often require steep Trendelenburg positioning to improve pelvic exposure. Trendelenburg position classically involves a head-down tilt moving abdominal viscera cephalad thereby improving pelvic access but increasing diaphragmatic elevation, airway pressures and venous congestion. Additionally, Lithotomy position may also be indicated for certain procedures.

Pneumoperitoneum and positional changes produce predictable cardiopulmonary and neurophysiological effects that must be anticipated and managed **(Table 1)**.

Preoperative Assessment and Optimization

- A thorough Pre-anesthesia checkup (PAC)
    - History: Complete history to be taken to rule out any systemic illness, H/O of allergies, previous anesthesia exposure, postoperative nausea vomiting, exercise tolerance

TABLE 1: Physiological effects of pneumoperitoneum and Trendelenburg.

System	*Effect*	*Anesthetic management*
Cardiovascular	↑ SVR, ↑ afterload, ↓ venous return → may ↓ CO	Maintain normovolemia; titrate insufflation pressure; vasopressors if needed
Respiratory	↓ FRC & compliance, ↑ airway pressures, ↑ $PaCO_2$	Controlled ventilation; increase minute ventilation; monitor $EtCO_2$ and arterial blood gas as required
Renal	↓ renal perfusion and urine output	Maintain MAP and euvolemia; minimize prolonged high insufflation pressures
Neurological	↑ ICP & IOP with head-down tilt	Avoid hypercapnia; limit degree/ duration of Trendelenburg when possible

TABLE 2: Key preoperative considerations.

Domain	*Action/Consideration*
Cardiovascular	Assess ischemic heart disease, optimize medications, consider cardiology review if unstable
Respiratory	Optimize COPD/asthma; smoking cessation; deep breathing exercises, chest physiotherapy if needed
Airway	Identify predictors of difficult intubation; plan equipment and personnel
Hematology/ Metabolic	Detect and correct anemia; manage diabetes and electrolytes

- Examination: Vitals, weight, BMI, difficult airway predictors
- Preoperative investigations: CBC, LFT, KFT, coagulation profile, Thyroid profile (wherever indicated), Type and screen, viral markers. ECG, blood crossmatch if required
- INFORMED CONSENT for anesthesia is a MUST.

On the basis of PAC findings preoperative optimization is done which includes treating active respiratory infection, controlling blood pressure, blood sugar, and correcting anemia where feasible **(Table 2)**.

Morbid obesity and COPD are common pre-existing conditions complicating ventilation and gas exchange during the surgery.

On the day of surgery:

- Pt. should be fasting for minimum 6–8 hours (clear fluids – water/apple juice/coconut water can be allowed up to 2 hours prior to surgery. Carbohydrate rich drink 2 hours prior to surgery leads to a better hemodynamic stability intraoperatively.

- All antihypertensives except for Angiotensin 2 receptor blockers (e.g., Losartan) should be continued till morning of surgery
- Oral hypoglycemics/Insulin to be discontinued on the morning of surgery. FBS, S. electrolytes to be done on the morning of surgery.
- Patients on anticoagulants, e.g., Clopidogrel, should stop them 5–7 days prior to surgery with consultation of the cardiologist. Tab. Ecosprin 75 mg can be continued till the day of surgery.

ANESTHETIC TECHNIQUE AND INTRAOPERATIVE MANAGEMENT

General anesthesia with endotracheal intubation and controlled ventilation remains the standard for most procedures. Minor procedures not requiring extreme position can also be done with supraglottic airway like Proseal LMA/I gel with controlled ventilation. TIVA (propofol/remifentanil) or volatile-based maintenance are both appropriate; choice depends on patient factors and surgical duration. Nitrous oxide is commonly avoided in laparoscopy to prevent bowel distension. Spinal anesthesia can be used as an adjunct in major procedures especially in obese population as it contracts the gut, thereby giving a better field of vision.

Monitoring and Special Considerations

- Standard ASA monitoring: ECG, NIBP, SpO_2, capnography and temperature is mandatory. Consider arterial line for major or prolonged cases.
- Vigilance for subcutaneous emphysema (rising $EtCO_2$).
- DVT pump to be applied in surgeries expected to last >2 hours
- Shoulder support is mandatory whenever steep Trendelenburg position is expected
- All the pressure points to be padded adequately
- A good IV line is a MUST
- Slow insufflation with IAP between 12–15 mm Hg, (chances of bradycardia at due to stretching of peritoneum at the initiation of pneumoperitoneum)
- Vigilance during insertion of trocar for any intra-abdominal injury
- Watch for the blood loss and urine output

Ventilation Strategy

Lung-protective ventilation principles are used: Low tidal volumes (6–8 $mL \cdot kg^{-1}$ ideal body weight), appropriate PEEP and increased minute ventilation to maintain normocapnia during CO_2 absorption.

Keep an eye for increase in airway pressures intraoperatively, which can be due to the steep Trendelenburg position/pneumoperitoneum/kinking of ETT/bronchospasm/endobronchial migration of ETT.

Hemodynamic Management

Maintain euvolemia; treat hypotension with fluids and vasopressors as required. Avoid excessive positive pressure ventilation that may further reduce venous return.

Analgesia and Antiemesis

Multimodal analgesia reduces opioid requirements: paracetamol, NSAIDs, regional blocks (e.g., transversus abdominis plane or port-site infiltration) and consideration of adjuncts such as ketamine or alpha-2 agonists.

Laparoscopic procedures have a higher incidence of postoperative nausea vomiting compared to open procedures. Prophylactic antiemetics along with nonusage of nitrous oxide reduces the incidence **(Table 3)**.

Postoperative Management and ERAS Integration

Early mobilization, multimodal analgesia, minimizing drains and early oral intake are ERAS principles that apply to laparoscopic gynecology and improve outcomes.

The Anesthesiologist: A Silent Partner in Success

An anesthesiologist integrates physiology, pharmacology and perioperative principles to facilitate surgery while maintaining patient safety making best operative conditions available to the surgeon. Incorporating ERAS (Enhanced Recovery After Surgery) measures, optimizing ventilation and

TABLE 3: Common anaesthetic complications and management.

Complication	*Mechanism/Cause*	*Immediate management*
Hypercarbia	CO_2 absorption from pneumoperitoneum	Increase minute ventilation; reduce insufflation pressure; consider ABG if required
Hypotension	Decreased venous return, vasodilation	Bolus crystalloid; vasopressor (phenylephrine/ephedrine)
Bradycardia/asystole	Vagal reflexes during insufflation or peritoneal stretch	Stop insufflation; atropine; abdomen to be deflated, slow reinflation, intra-abdominal pressures (12–15 mm Hg)
Subcutaneous emphysema	Gas tracking into tissue planes	Reduce insufflation pressure; monitor airway and $EtCO_2$; CT if extensive
Nerve injury	Inadequate padding of pressure points, hyper extension of joints (M/C – common peroneal nerve)	All the pressure points should be padded adequately, low lithotomy whenever possible

hemodynamics and preventing complications makes an anesthesiologist indispensable for a good surgical outcome.

KEY POINTS

- Anesthesia is integral to laparoscopic gynecological surgery, ensuring patient safety and optimal surgical conditions.
- Pneumoperitoneum and steep Trendelenburg position cause predictable cardiovascular and respiratory changes that must be anticipated.
- Preoperative optimization of comorbidities (especially obesity, COPD, cardiovascular disease) improves intraoperative stability.
- General anesthesia with controlled ventilation remains standard; TIVA and multimodal analgesia enhance recovery.
- Continuous capnography, vigilance for rising airway pressures, and early detection of hypercarbia or hypotension are vital.
- Enhanced Recovery After Surgery (ERAS) principles—early mobilization, multimodal analgesia, and minimal drains—shorten recovery time.
- The anesthesiologist's coordination of pre-, intra-, and postoperative care determines the quality of surgical outcomes, making them a true partner in surgical success.

SUGGESTED READING

1. Association of Anaesthetists of Great Britain and Ireland (AAGBI). Perioperative care of adult patients undergoing laparoscopic surgery. Anaesthesia. 2019;74(8):1105-16.
2. Dubey N, Bellamy F. Systematic review and network meta-analysis of intraperitoneal local anaesthetics for laparoscopic abdominal surgery. Br J Anaesth. 2024;132:562-74.
3. ERAS® Society. Guidelines for pre- and intra-operative care in gynecologic/oncology surgery: Part I. Stockholm: ERAS® Society; 2019.
4. Finkelstein J, Eckersberge E, Sadri H, Taneja SS, Lepor H, Djavan B. Open versus laparoscopic versus robotic assisted laparoscopic prostatectomy: The European and US Experience. Rev Urol. 2010;12(1):35-43.
5. Gupta R, Sharma R. Anaesthesia for laparoscopic gynaecological surgery: physiological changes and anaesthetic considerations. Indian J Anaesth. 2019;63(9):731-8.
6. Hanly EJ, Talamini MA. Robotic abdominal surgery. Am J Surg. 2004;188(4A Suppl):19S-26S.
7. Hirsch M, Tariq L, Duffy JM. Effect of local anaesthetics on postoperative pain after laparoscopic gynaecological procedures: systematic review. J Minim Invasive Gynecol. 2021;28(10):1689-98.
8. Jenkins ES, Nelson G. Enhanced recovery after surgery (ERAS) guided gynaecologic pathways: outcomes and implementation. Gynecol Oncol Rep. 2024;55:101510.
9. Mack MJ. Minimally invasive and robotic surgery. JAMA. 2001;285(5):568-72.
10. Major AL, et al. Gynecological Laparoscopic Surgeries under Spinal Anaesthesia: feasibility and outcomes. J Clin Anaesth. 2024; (prospective cohort study).

11. McMahon AJ. Cardiopulmonary effects of laparoscopic surgery. Br J Anaesth. 1993;71(4):459-63.
12. Miller RD, Cohen NH, Eriksson LI, Fleisher LA, Wiener-Kronish JP, Young WL. Miller's Anaesthesia, 9th edition. Amsterdam: Elsevier; 2020.
13. Morgan GE, Mikhail MS, Murray MJ. Clinical Anaesthesiology, 6th edition. New York: McGraw-Hill; 2018.
14. Ostermann M, Auzinger G, Grocott M, Morton-Bailey V, Raphael J, Shaw AD, et al. Perioperative fluid management: evidence-based recommendations. Br J Anaesth. 2024;133(6):1263-75.
15. Radkowski P. Optimizing Anaesthetic Management for Laparoscopic Surgery. J Perioper Med. 2024; (review article).
16. Weinberg L, Rao S, Escobar PF. Robotic surgery in gynaecology: an updated systemic review. Obstet Gynecol Int. 2011;2011:852061.

4 CHAPTER

Optimizing Complex Bladder Dissection in Scarred Uterus

Sejal Naik, Ritu Jain, Aditi Modi

When the canvas is scarred, it is the surgical artist who makes all the difference!!

INTRODUCTION

In ObGyn, safe bladder dissection in a scarred uterus is a critical concern, especially in patients with history of prior caesarean sections or other pelvic surgeries. Scar tissue can distort normal anatomy, increase the risk of bladder and ureter injury, prolong operating time, increase the morbidity, and recovery at the same time, compromise results. Guidelines focus on meticulous preoperative assessment, strategic surgical techniques, and high intra- and postoperative vigilance.

PREOPERATIVE ASSESSMENT AND PLANNING

- *Detailed History and Risk Assessment:* Review patient's full surgical history, inclusive of number and type of previous caesarean sections or other pelvic surgeries. A history of one or more cesarean deliveries is a significant risk factor for dense bladder adhesions.
- *Imaging studies:* In cases of previous cesarean sections and pelvic surgeries, preoperative ultrasound **(Fig. 1)** can help identify bladder's upper limit,

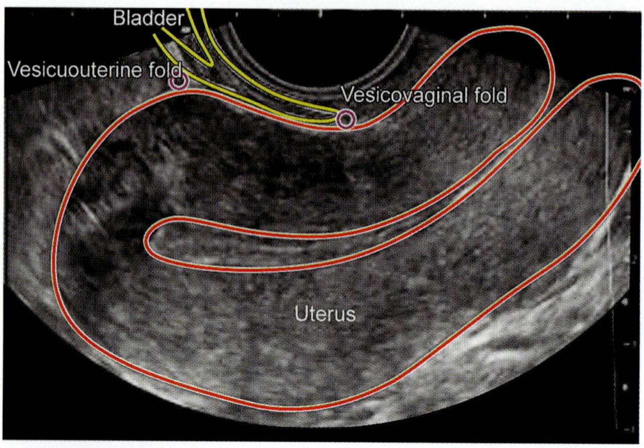

Fig. 1: Bladder limit delineation on preoperative USG.
Courtesy: https://doi.org/10.1002/uog.29128

particularly if it sits high on the uterus due to previous surgery. This helps surgeons modify abdominal entry point, to enter peritoneum higher to avoid injury. "Sliding sign" in ultrasound is useful for diagnosing intra-abdominal adhesion. In absence of adhesion, during deep breathing the uterus will slide below parietal fascia whereas in severe adhesion, this sliding is absent.

- *Informed consent:* In high-risk cases, during informed consent process, discussion of potential for difficult dissection and increased risk of urological tract injuries with patients is important.
- *Anticipatory Operative Preparedness:* Being prepared for intraoperative injuries is helpful. A multidisciplinary team with stand-by extra surgical hands and required OT instruments and disposables is advisable. Given the complexity of such cases with extensive scarring, such procedures should be performed by experienced surgeons with specific training in advanced surgical techniques.

STRATEGIC SURGICAL TECHNIQUES

- *Urinary catheterization:* While routinely performed, it does not fully prevent injury. The use of a catheter allows for bladder decompression.
- *Controlled Bladder filling:* In few TLH cases, intraoperative filling-up of bladder with normal saline prior to adhesion dissection would reduce chances of injury by helping to delineate its margins.
- *Sharp Vs Blunt Dissection:* When dense adhesions are present, sharp dissection with controlled and careful movements is often preferred over blunt dissection, which can lead to inadvertent bladder damage. Keeping the dissecting instrument's tip close to uterine serosa helps maintain planes.
- *Traction and Counter-Traction:* Safety lies in the hands of the surgeon. Judicious use of traction and counter-traction mechanisms helps maintain tension on tissues, which clarifies surgical planes. One can use the cervical cup to demarcate the lower limit of the bladder dissection.
- *Judicious Usage of Energy Sources:* Adhere to principle of using energy sources judiciously and for short bursts, to avoid thermal injury. Consider using ultrasonic energy, which reduces thermal spread. Avoid excessive electrocautery near the bladder to prevent thermal necrosis **(Fig. 2)** and delayed complications like vesicovaginal fistula
- *Manage bleeding:* Ligation of ascending uterine blood supply prior to addressing difficult bladder flap is useful. Control bleeding early in dissection to prevent blood from staining the tissues, which can obscurc anatomical planes and increase difficulty of dissection. Uterine vessels can be ligated with sutures instead of cauterization when bladder is adherent.

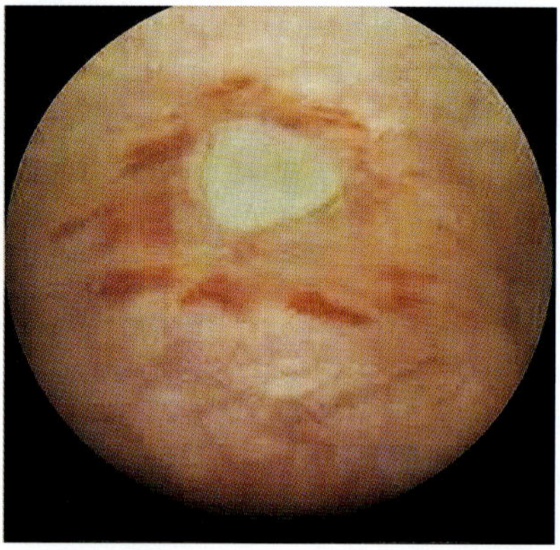

Fig. 2: Thermal bladder injury on cystoscopy.
Courtesy: https://doi.org/10.33696/Gynaecology.6.079

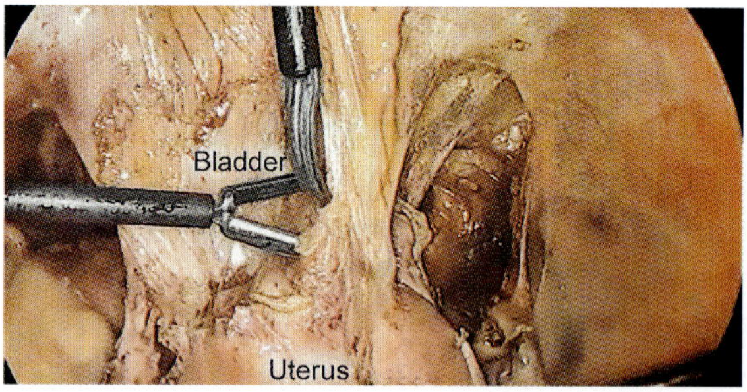

Fig. 3: Lateral approach for bladder dissection (SpringerLink).

PROCEDURE-SPECIFIC SURGICAL TECHNIQUES

LAVH/ TLH/ Robotic Hysterectomy/ vNOTES:

- *Transvaginal lateral intervention in LAVH:* Lateral window of vesicocervical space are created; an index finger is swept medially to define margin of midline vesicocervical adhesions. Under direct vision and finger guidance, the dense adhesions dissected safely. Subsequently, the bladder is pushed gently aside to prevent its tearing or injury.
- Low And Lateral Approach to identify clean plane for dissection described by Seth S et al., for hysterectomy in patients with Previous CS. In laparoscopy, once the uterine vascular bundle is identified, dissection proceeds just above these vessels to lateral cervical margins. The midline adhesions are separated later, under better visualization **(Fig. 3)**.
- Rao and Kade also introduced a six-step laparoscopic technique for dissecting a central uterine band in a ventrofixed uterus, aiming to minimize injury to adjacent structures during repeat cesarean sections and hysterectomy **(Fig. 4)**:

  Step 1: Dissect the left round ligament; this dissection should be parallel and above this ligament.

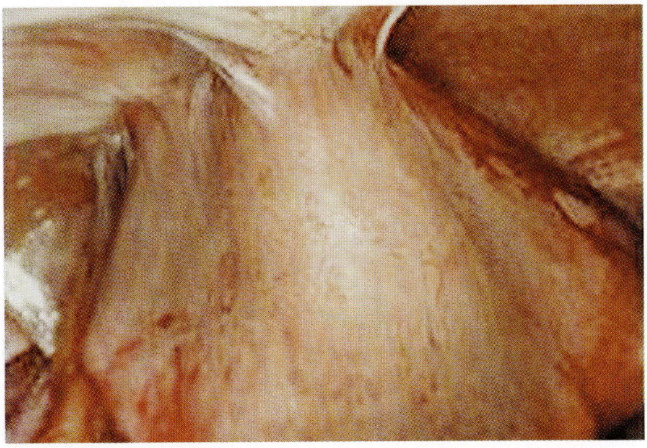

Fig. 4: Ventrofixed uterus.

Step 2: Identify the left uterine artery.
Step 3: Dissect the right round ligament.
Step 4: Identify the right uterine artery.
Step 5: Dissect the avascular space between the bladder and central uterine band bilaterally.
Step 6: Separate the central uterine adhesion band from the anterior abdominal wall (parietal peritoneum).

- HUBB (Hung Up the Bladder Bypass) technique: A laparoscopic method for dissecting a highly adherent bladder in hysterectomies. Steps of HUBB technique:
  - Identify and locate uterine artery and its position.
  - Create a retrovesical lower uterine segment bypass (**Fig. 5A**)
  - Create a "Hung Up the Bladder Bypass": A second bypass, which allows for complete bladder dissection **(Fig. 5B)**
  - Perform Adhesiolysis and Leak Test: Separate any adhesions and perform a leak test to ensure Urinary tract integrity.

  Benefits HUBB technique:
  - voids Complications: It minimizes risk of bladder injury,
  - Improves Dissection: Provides clearer and more defined dissection space
  - Facilitates Repair: It helps with patient orientation for a potential repair if any damage does occur.
- Comprehensive Canopy Concept, "The 3 Step Technique": To address the challenges beyond conventional lateral approach for bladder dissection, Nutan et al. introduced a comprehensive canopy concept which unfolds in three distinct steps **(Figs. 6A to F)**
  - The initial step involves posterior approach to uterine artery dissection, coagulation, and section.
  - Subsequently, creation of bladder canopy, strategically addressing varying levels of adherence.

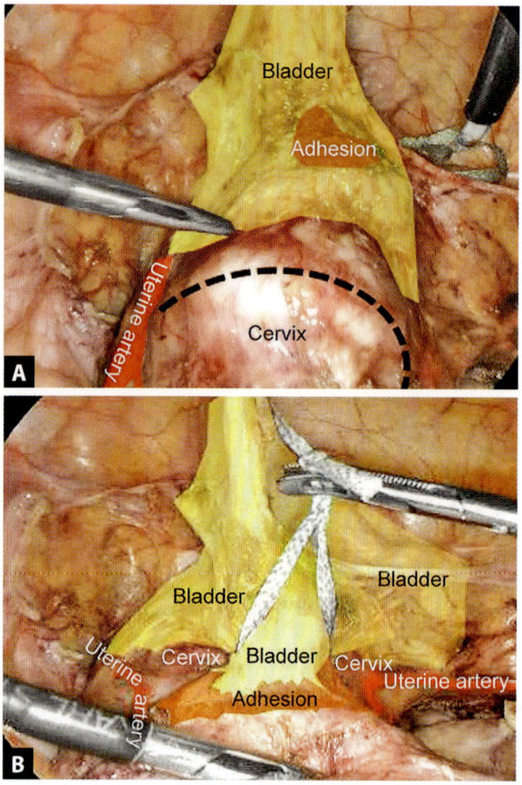

Figs. 5A and B: (A) Locating uterine vessels and start creating retrovesical LUS Bypass; and (B) Creating hung up blabber bypass.

  - Introduced recently, an anterior approach to uterine artery dissection and coagulation. This includes reaching the contralateral uterine artery by side of the manipulator cup rim in one single sweep.
- *Head-on and Reverse Dissection:* Studies have indicated that while lateral approach was adequate in most cases of vNOTES, it did not allow access to peritoneal cavity when there were significant adhesions at vesicouterine peritoneum. In these circumstances, direct dissection of adhesions was necessary. For Laparoscopic or Robotic Hysterectomies, "head-on" approach involves superior-to-inferior dissection. A "reverse vesicouterine fold dissection" starts dissection from an inferior, less-adherent plane and proceeds superiorly **(Figs. 7 and 8)**. Both techniques are used to find correct anatomical plane and safely mobilize bladder. Working from lateral to medial, utilizing uterine manipulator with cervical delineation and backfilling bladder, also helps in RH and TLH.
- Sunkara et al. described Four Steps of Difficult bladder dissection:
  - Backfilling bladder to delineate bladder boundaries and avoid inadvertent injury.

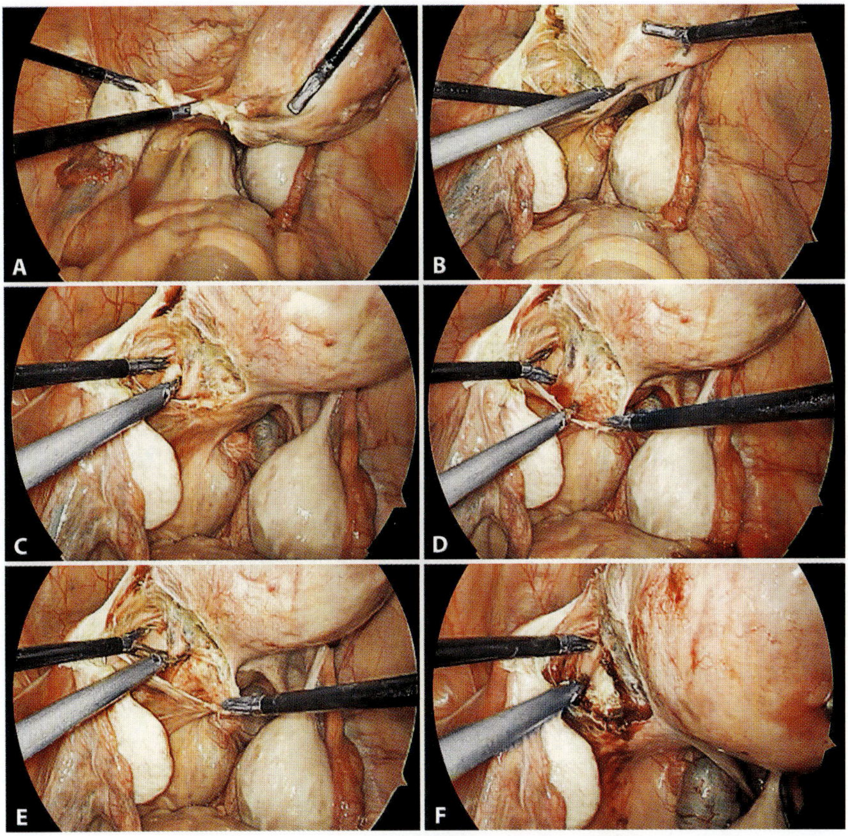

Figs. 6A to F: Comprehensive Canopy Concept, "The 3 Step Technique".

- Lateral approach, for Adhesiolysis, followed by cephalad dissection towards bladder dome.
- Lateralization of uterine arteries prior to bladder dissection.
- Create posterior colpotomy and carry incision anteriorly to help delineate normal anatomical markers.

INTRA- AND POSTOPERATIVE TOOLS AND VIGILANCE

- *Intraoperative identification:* Constantly be aware of key landmarks. The uterine sound, catheter bulb, cervical cup, or uterine manipulator can help identify uterine and bladder limits to minimize risk of bladder injury, enhance visualization and precision during dissection. Additionally.
- *Retrograde Cystoinflation:* In RCT's, these techniques have shown significant reduction in bladder injury rates in high-risk patients, during dissection. Intraoperative bladder distension with Saline (Cystoinflation), Methylene Blue Dye or ICG dye using near-infrared technology can help delineate boundaries and extent, improving visualization.

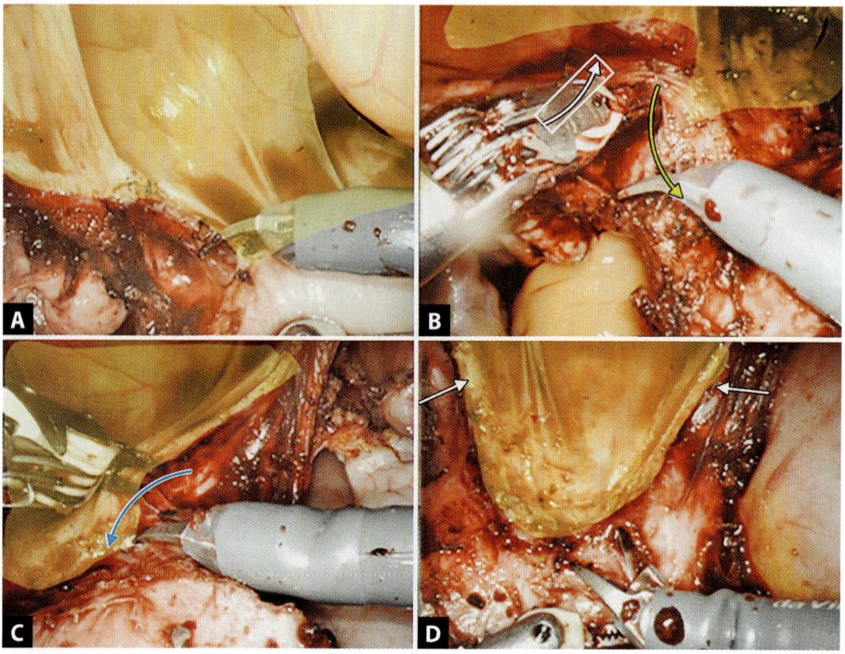

Figs. 7A to D: Reverse bladder dissection with Head-on Approach. (A) Adherent Bladder at LUS; (B) Space beneath adherent bladder in LUS on left; (C) Space beneath adherent bladder in LUS on right; and (D) Head-on Approach of central adhesion, following bilateral reverse dissection.

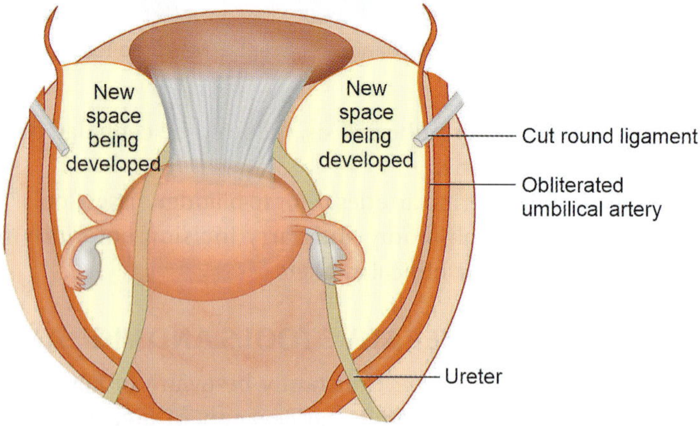

Fig. 8: Neo Space Creation by Reverse Vesicouterine Fold Dissection Technique. Creation of New Space in Vesicovaginal area, using blunt sweeping motion from inferior-to-superior direction, facilitates hysterectomy in patients with severe anterior cul-de-sac adhesions from prior caesarean deliveries or other surgeries.

- *Integrity Confirmation:* At conclusion of dissection, or if an injury is suspected, fill the bladder with sterile fluid or methylene blue dye to check for any leaks. Cystoscopy may also be performed.

- *Postoperative care:* In cases of bladder repair, extended catheterization for 10–14 days is typically recommended.
- *Postoperative Urine Retention:* Difficult bladder dissection and manipulation can lead to postoperative urine retention. Vigilant watch is required.

CONCLUSION

Safe bladder dissection in a scarred uterus requires a multifaceted approach that combines meticulous preoperative assessment, strategic surgical techniques, and high intraoperative vigilance. By understanding the patient's surgical history, utilizing imaging studies, and employing techniques such as sharp dissection, traction and counter-traction, controlled bladder filling, and judicious energy use, surgeons can minimize the risk of bladder injury. Surgical skills and technique are more important than instruments. Do not leave in doubt, Intraoperative tools like retrograde cystoinflation and cystoscopy can aid in identifying and repairing injuries. By adopting these strategies, surgeons can improve patient outcomes, reduce morbidity, and ensure a successful surgical experience. Ultimately, a well-planned and executed approach to bladder dissection in a scarred uterus is crucial for optimizing patient care and minimizing complications.

KEY POINTS

- Safe bladder dissection in a scarred uterus requires a multifaceted approach that combines meticulous preoperative assessment, strategic surgical techniques, and high intraoperative vigilance along with postoperative follow up.
- Understanding the patient's surgical history, utilizing imaging studies, and employing techniques such as sharp dissection, traction and counter-traction, controlled bladder filling, and judicious energy use, minimizes the risk of bladder injury.
- Surgical skills and technique are more important than instruments.
- Do not leave in doubt, Intraoperative tools like retrograde cystoinflation and cystoscopy can aid in identifying and repairing injuries.

SUGGESTED READING

1. Arcieri M, Cuman M, Restaino S, Tius V, Cianci S, Ronsini C, et al. Exploring Urinary Tract Injuries in Gynaecological Surgery: Current Insights and Future Directions. Healthcare. 2025;13(15):1780.
2. Baron J, Tirosh D, Mastrolia SA, Ben-Haroush Y, Schwartz S, Kerner Y, et al. Sliding sign in third-trimester sonographic evaluation of intra-abdominal adhesions in women undergoing repeat Cesarean section: A novel technique. Ultrasound Obstet Gynecol. 2018;52:662-5.
3. Caplan M, Misal M. Key techniques for difficult bladder dissection during robotic assisted total laparoscopic hysterectomy. Am J Obstet Gynaecol. 2024;230(4):S1297.

4. Chang WC, Hsu WC, Sheu BC, Huang SC, Torng PL, Chang DY. Minimizing bladder injury in laparoscopically assisted vaginal hysterectomy among women with previous caesarean sections. Surg Endosc. 2008;22:171-6.
5. Dwivedi A, Dave A, Thora A, Pandit M, Lakhra A. A prospective cohort study to determine effectiveness of cystoinflation to prevent bladder injury in women with previous caesarean section. Int J Reprod Contracept Obstetr Gynaecol. 2025;14(8):2579-84.
6. Fangmann LC, Henrich W, Hinkson L. Assessment of the urinary bladder prior to caesarean delivery in women with multiple abdominal scars through operation table ultrasonography: a case report. AJOG Glob Rep. 2023;3(1):100138.
7. Hafeez R, khan U. (2008) A Review Study of Bladder Injury in Laparoscopy Assisted Vaginal Hysterectomy. [online] Available from https://www.semanticscholar.org/paper/A-Review-Study-of-Bladder-Injury-in-Laparoscopy/a08ed0712491fe8410801be91b181ef73bbf5b35. [Last accessed January, 2026].
8. Jain N. 12216 The 3-Step: Comprehensive Canopy Concept Versus Lateral Approach of Bladder Dissection in TLH With Previous Caesarean Sections. J Minim Invasive Gynaecol. 31(11):S139.
9. Nezhat C, Vu M, Vang N, Tombash E, Nezhat A. Hysterectomy in patients with history of prior caesarean delivery: A reverse dissection technique for vesicouterine adhesions. OBG Manag. 2019;31(11):38-42.
10. Rao T, Kade S. Ventrofixed uterus: unfreezing the uterus in 6 standardized steps. J Gynecol Surg. 2023;39:220-1.
11. Saaqib S, Iqbal A, Naheed M, Saeed T, Khalid M. A randomized controlled trial of cystoinflation to prevent bladder injury in the adhesive disease of multiple caesarean sections. Sci Rep. 2020;10(1):15297.
12. Shikha S, Arun N. Preventing Bladder Injury at Hysterectomy in Post-Caesareans. J Gynecol Women's Health. 2017;3(2):555610.
13. Sinha R, Rupa B, Peddappolla S. Redefining Bladder Dissection in Robotic Hysterectomy with Previous Caesarean Section: A "Head-On Approach". Cureus. 2025;17(8):e90280.
14. Sunkara S, Koythong T, Nijjar JB, Chohan L. Approach to Difficult Bladder Dissection during Laparoscopic Hysterectomy. J Minim Invasive Gynaecol. 2020;27(7):S103.
15. Tamate M, Matsuura M, Wada N, Adachi T, Yorozu K, Arimoto C, et al. Laparoscopic retro vesical lower uterine segment bypass for hysterectomy with previous caesarean section: Hung Up the Bladder Bypass (HUBB) technique. J Gynecol Obstet Hum Reprod. 2023;52(8):102629.
16. Tantitamit T, Temtanakitpaisan T, Lee CL. Bladder safety during natural orifice transluminal endoscopic surgery hysterectomy in patients with extensive vesicouterine adhesion. Gynecol Minim Invasive Ther. 2019;8:129-31.
17. Zelivianskaia AS, Bradley SE, Morozov VV. Best practices for repair of iatrogenic bladder injury. AJOG Glob Rep. 2022;2(3):100062.

5 CHAPTER

Tackling the Uterine Artery in Gynecological Endoscopy: Why, When, How?

Sejal Naik, Ritu Jain

INTRODUCTION

The uterine artery plays a crucial role in uterine vascular supply and is a key anatomical and functional structure in gynecological endoscopy. Mastering uterine artery control enables gynecologic surgeons to perform minimally invasive surgeries more safely and effectively, especially in procedures with high bleeding risk such as laparoscopic hysterectomy, myomectomy, endometriosis excision, and oncological dissections.

This chapter discusses the indications, rationale, laparoscopic technique, timing, precautions, and clinical implications of uterine artery ligation or devascularization in gynecological endoscopy.

ANATOMICAL OVERVIEW ORIGIN: INTERNAL ILIAC ARTERY (ANTERIOR DIVISION) (FIG. 1)

- *Course:* Medial to the pelvic sidewall, passing over the ureter ("water under the bridge"), entering the uterus at the level of the isthmus.
- *Branches:* Ascending and descending uterine branches, cervical and vaginal branches
- *Ureteric relation:* The ureter passes just beneath the uterine artery ~1.5 cm lateral to the cervix, placing it at high risk during surgery.

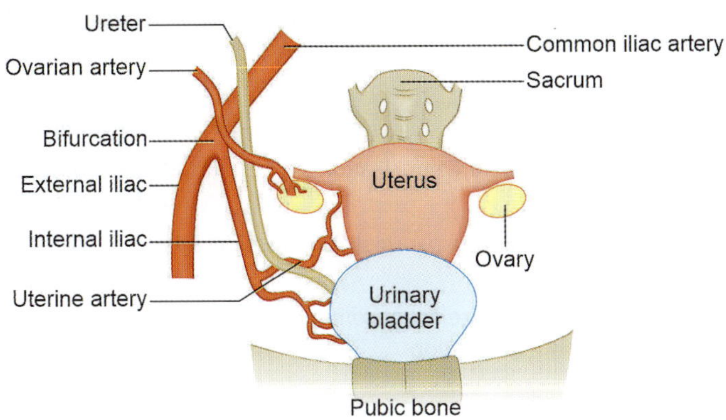

Fig. 1: Anatomical overview of origin and course of uterine artery.

WHY TACKLE THE UTERINE ARTERY?

- *Hemostasis:* Major indication in myomectomy, adenomyosis, TLH. Reduces intraoperative blood loss by 50–60%.
- *Volume Reduction:* Large fibroids or bulky uteri shrink and become more manageable after devascularization.
- *Visibility and Surgical Ease:* Bloodless field improve precision, reduces operative time.
- *Fertility-Sparing Alternative:* In select cases of AUB, laparoscopic bilateral uterine artery ligation (LUAL) can avoid hysterectomy.

WHEN TO TACKLE THE UTERINE ARTERY: CLINICAL SITUATIONS WHERE UTERINE ARTERY LIGATION IS NEEDED

See **Figure 2** and **Tables 1 and 2**.

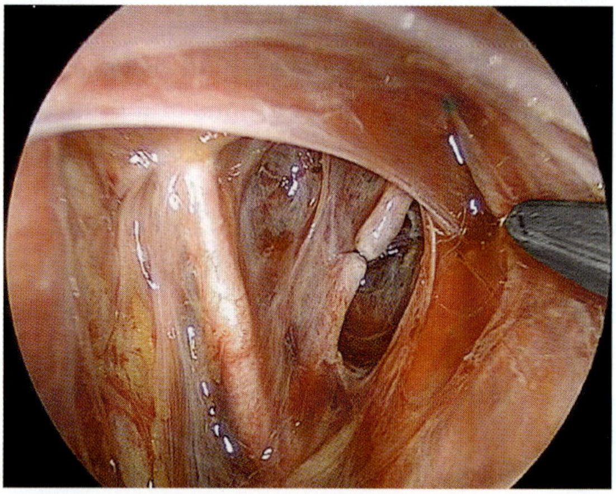

Fig. 2: Ligation of uterine artery.

TABLE 1: Clinical scenarios requiring uterine artery ligation.

Procedure	*Preferred timing*	*Why*
Total Laparoscopic Hysterectomy	Early	Reduces bleeding before uterine pedicles
Myomectomy	Before enucleation	Shrinks fibroids, cleaner field
Endometriosis excision	Before parametrial dissection	Prevents bleeding from deep implants
Oncology Cases	Before or concomitant during dissection	Hemorrhage control

CONTRAINDICATIONS

TABLE 2: Contraindications.

Absolute	*Relative*
Suspicion of pelvic arteriovenous malformation	Severe pelvic adhesions or distorted anatomy
	Coagulopathy or bleeding disorders

HOW: LAPAROSCOPIC UTERINE ARTERY CONTROL—STEP BY STEP (TABLES 3 AND 4)

Approach: Transperitoneal

Devices: Bipolar, vessel sealer (LigaSure, ENSEAL), laparoscopic clips Ports: 10 mm umbilical, 5 mm lateral

1. Identify Pelvic Landmarks Round ligament, Infundibulopelvic (IP) ligament, Ureter.
2. Open Broad Ligament Incise anterior leaf of the broad ligament. Create a window medial to IP ligament and lateral to ureter.
3. Identify the Uterine Artery Trace its origin from the internal iliac artery. Follow its path medially where it crosses over the ureter.

TABLE 3: Key anatomical considerations.

Structure	*Relevance*
Uterine artery	Supplies uterus; crosses over ureter
Ureter	Under uterine artery ("water under the bridge")
Internal iliac artery Uterine Isthmus	Source of uterine artery (Anterior Division) Entry point of uterine artery into uterus
Broad ligament window	Access to retroperitoneal space for vessel isolation

TABLE 4: Comparison of techniques.

Method	*Approach*	*Indications*	*Advantages*	*Disadvantages*
Laparoscopic Ligation	Endoscopic	TLH, myomectomy	Visual control, precise, safe	Requires advanced skills
Vaginal Ligation	Blind	PPH, VH	Rapid, accessible	Higher risk of ureter injury
Embolization (UAE)	Percutaneous Radiologic	Fibroids, AVM, PPH	Minimally invasive, fertility-preserving	Expensive, Post-embolization syndrome, radiation exposure

4. Skeletonize the Vessel Dissect perivascular tissue to expose the artery fully. Protect nearby veins and ureter.
5. Coagulate and Divide **(Fig. 3)**
6. Use bipolar or energy device to coagulate ~1.5–2 cm from the uterus. Optionally place laparoscopic clip before division **(Fig. 4)**, or temporary shoe lace knot can also be applied **(Figs. 5A and B)**

COMMON ERRORS TO AVOID

- Coagulating uterine artery without skeletonization
- Blind application of clips or energy near ureter
- Attempting ligation in distorted anatomy without ureter identification
- Assuming hemostasis without post-coagulation inspection
- Over dissection causing avulsion or tear in vessel

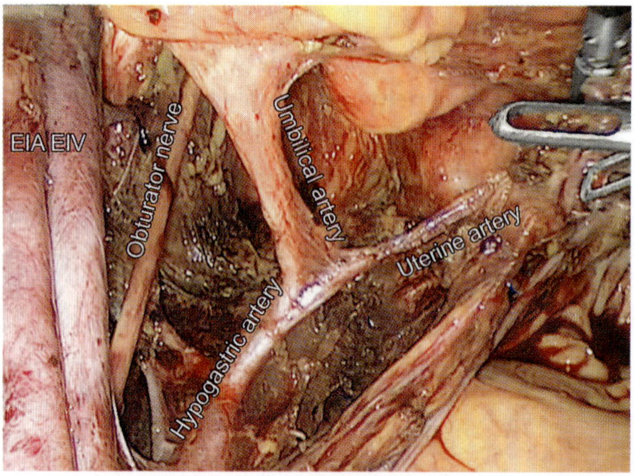

Fig. 3: Uterine artery at origin—dissection and coagulation.

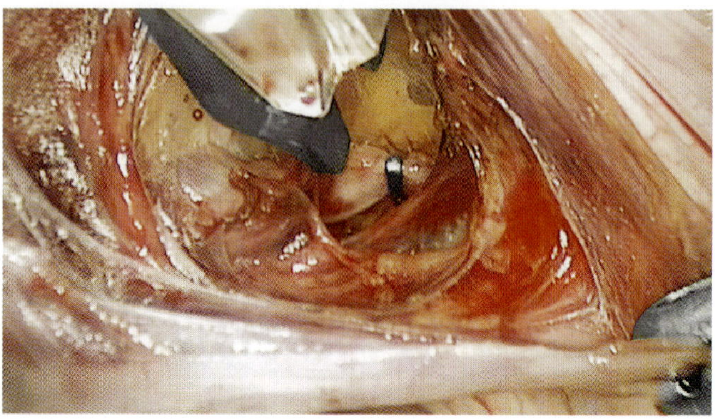

Fig. 4: Laparoscopic view of the clip located at the uterine artery.

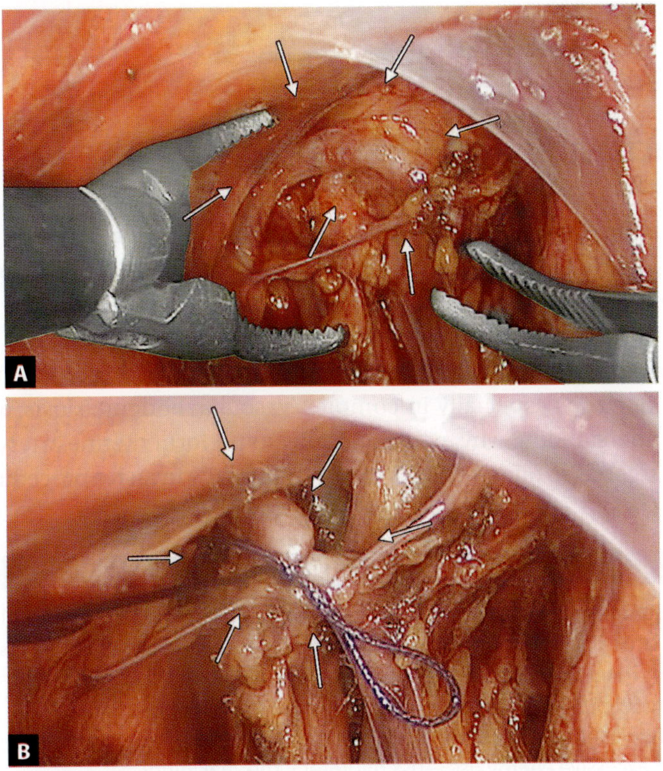

Figs. 5A and B: Temporary uterine artery ligation during the surgical procedure. (A) The right uterine artery was identified and isolated from the anterior branch of the internal iliac artery; and (B) The right uterine artery was ligated with a multifilament suture. The arrow shows the right uterine artery.

PRECAUTIONS AND SAFETY TIPS TO AVOID URETERIC INJURY

1. Always visualize ureter before vessel coagulation.
2. Keep coagulation lateral to ureteric path.
3. Avoid thermal spread—use brief, low-energy bursts.
4. Use sharp dissection in dense adhesions.
5. In difficult anatomy, clip without dividing the artery.
6. Avoid excessive traction on bladder pillar.
7. Consider prophylactic stenting in complex cases

KEY ANATOMICAL POINTS

Complications to Watch For:

1. Ureteric injury—thermal, transection, or clip entrapment

2. Vessel avulsion or bleeding
3. Incomplete devascularization
4. Hematoma formation

CONCLUSION

Tackling the uterine artery is a critical step and a valuable safety increasing skill in various gynecological procedures. A thorough understanding of pelvic anatomy, particularly the course of the ureter and internal iliac branches, is essential.

Laparoscopic ligation provides a minimally invasive, effective method for devascularizing the uterus, reducing surgical blood loss and expanding surgical horizons especially in complex/vascular/endometriosis/oncology cases. Understanding why, when and how to perform uterine artery control allows surgeons to offer fertility-sparing, minimally invasive procedures with confidence.

KEY POINTS

- The uterine artery is best tackled early in cases with anticipated heavy bleeding (e.g., large fibroids, TLH), enabling bloodless surgery and better outcomes.
- Always identify and protect the ureter before any vessel handling.
- Laparoscopic approach offers visual clarity and precise dissection.
- Use bipolar or clips, depending on anatomy, resource availability, and surgeon skill.
- Avoid excessive energy use—risk of ureteric thermal injury
- Embolization is an alternative but has limitations.
- Mastery of pelvic anatomy is critical for safe uterine artery control.

SUGGESTED READING

1. AAGL. Laparoscopic hysterectomy: practice guidelines. J Minim Invasive Gynecol. 2021.
2. Committee on Practice Bulletins—Gynecology. ACOG. Management of Abnormal Uterine Bleeding. Practice Bulletin No. 128. Obstet Gynecol. 2012;120(1):197-206.
3. Dubuisson JB, et al. Laparoscopic ligation of uterine arteries in fibroid treatment. Obstet Gynecol. 1995.
4. Nezhat C. Pelvic anatomy and uterine artery control. Operative Gynecol Endosc. 2020.
5. Pisat S, van Herendael BJ. Temporary Ligation of the Uterine Artery at Its Origin Using a Removable "Shoelace" Knot. J Minim Invasive Gynecol. 2020;27(1):26.
6. Tulandi T. Techniques for uterine artery occlusion in myomectomy. Fertil Steril. 2012.

6 CHAPTER

Vaginal Vault Support during Total Laparoscopic Hysterectomy

Parul Kotadawala, Munjal Pandya

INTRODUCTION

Pelvic organ prolapse (POP) commonly occurs following childbirth or weakening of the pelvic floor. It can also develop after hysterectomy if the upper vaginal supports are not properly restored. When the uterosacral–cardinal ligament complex is not reattached, the vaginal vault can lose its support and gradually descend due to abdominal pressure. Reported rates of post-hysterectomy prolapse differ considerably—from less than 1% to over 40%—depending on surgical approach, follow-up period, and patient demographics.

As total laparoscopic hysterectomy (TLH) has become the standard treatment for benign uterine disorders, ensuring proper support of the vaginal apex during the procedure is essential to prevent later prolapse.

ANATOMICAL BASIS

Pelvic support is classically described using DeLancey's three-level model, which outlines the distinct structures maintaining vaginal integrity.

Level I: uterosacral-cardinal ligament complex, providing suspension of the vaginal apex.
Level II: paravaginal and connective-tissue attachments of the mid-vagina.
Level III: perineal body and distal muscular supports.

Damage to Level I structures during hysterectomy is the main factor contributing to vault prolapse. Additional factors—such as thermal injury, reduced blood flow, or excessive traction—can further compromise the apical support system. During TLH, precise identification of the uterosacral ligaments is essential because tactile feedback is limited and the ureters course closely lateral to the ligaments.

RISK FACTORS

Factors that increase the risk of vault prolapse include congenital or acquired connective-tissue weakness, multiple childbirths, menopause, obesity, chronic coughing or constipation, smoking, and a history of pelvic operations. Research shows that women who have undergone hysterectomy are several times more likely to require prolapse surgery later in life compared with those who have not. Among the contributing factors, failure to perform vault fixation during hysterectomy is the most preventable cause of post-hysterectomy vault prolapse.

RATIONALE FOR PROPHYLACTIC VAULT SUSPENSION

Securing the top of the vagina to the uterosacral and cardinal ligaments helps re-align the vaginal axis and reconstitute the primary apical support system. According to the joint guideline from RCOG and BSUG, surgeons should perform apical suspension during every hysterectomy for benign indications to minimize the risk of later vault prolapse.[2]

When vault suspension is not performed during the initial surgery, subsequent reconstructive procedures—whether abdominal, laparoscopic, or vaginal—tend to involve greater risks, higher costs, and an increased chance of recurrence. Consequently, incorporating vault support should be regarded as a routine and essential step in total laparoscopic hysterectomy rather than an optional addition.

TECHNIQUES FOR VAULT SUPPORT

Uterosacral Ligament Suspension

In uterosacral ligament suspension (USLS), the top of the vagina is reattached to the uterosacral ligaments on both sides to recreate natural apical support. In the laparoscopic "high" approach to USLS, as detailed by Ceccaroni et al., sutures are placed close to the sacral portion of the uterosacral ligaments. This positioning gives strong and long-lasting support while preserving the normal direction of the vaginal canal. In contrast, "low" USLS—performed near the ischial spine—is easier but has higher recurrence. Because the ureter passes only a short distance from the uterosacral ligaments, careful visualization and shallow suture placement are essential to avoid injury during suspension.

Delayed-absorbable monofilament or barbed sutures facilitate intracorporeal knot-tying and maintain tension without slippage. Clinical research indicates that this method results in less than a 5% recurrence rate, while maintaining vaginal dimensions and minimizing postoperative discomfort during intercourse.

McCall's Culdoplasty (Laparoscopic Adaptation)

McCall's Culdoplasty, first introduced in the late 1950s, involves closing the cul-de-sac (pouch of Douglas) by using the uterosacral ligaments to support and elevate the vaginal apex.

Laparoscopic adaptation replicates the same principle endoscopically, non-absorbable sutures are passed through the posterior vaginal angles and the uterosacral folds, drawing them together to close the cul-de-sac.

Recent research suggests that performing a laparoscopic McCall Culdoplasty during hysterectomy helps prevent vault descent and cuff complications, without notably increasing surgery time or blood loss. Long-term data show low recurrence and preserved coital function.

Sacrospinous Ligament Fixation

Sacrospinous ligament fixation (SSLF) may be carried out either vaginally or laparoscopically. In this technique, the top of the vagina is secured to the sacrospinous ligament, generally positioned a few centimeters from the ischial spine, using non-absorbable sutures. This approach gives firm support on one side but may slightly alter the vaginal orientation and occasionally lead to temporary discomfort in the buttock or sciatic region. Because of these drawbacks, SSLF is usually reserved for recurrent or complex prolapse rather than routine prophylaxis.

Round-Ligament Suspension

When the uterosacral ligaments are weak or inaccessible, the round ligaments can be used as an easier alternative for securing the vaginal vault. The round ligaments are identified near their uterine insertions and sutured to the corresponding vaginal angles using delayed-absorbable material. Even though round-ligament fixation provides less structural strength, short-term studies report satisfactory anatomical outcomes, little postoperative discomfort, and low complication rates. The technique avoids ureteric risk and is particularly useful in laparoscopic settings where rapid vault support is desired.

Combined Ligament Fixation

Combining several ligamentous structures—such as the uterosacral, cardinal, and round ligaments—can provide multidirectional support and distribute mechanical tension more evenly across the vault. Carlin et al. reported a recurrence rate below 1% when this technique was incorporated routinely into TLH. It is especially beneficial for women with pre-existing uterine descent or connective-tissue laxity.

OUTCOMES

Comprehensive reviews of multiple studies have shown that including an apical suspension step during hysterectomy markedly reduces the risk of future vault prolapse. Laparoscopic USLS and McCall Culdoplasty yield outcomes comparable to open or vaginal approaches with shorter hospital stay and faster recovery.

Studies suggest that prolapse develops in roughly one out of ten cases when the vaginal apex is not secured, whereas rates drop below two percent when fixation is performed. Economic analyses indicate that performing prophylactic apical fixation during the initial surgery decreases the likelihood and overall cost of future corrective operations.

Documented complications include temporary traction on the ureter, nerve-related buttock pain (particularly following sacrospinous fixation), and occasional cases of suture exposure or erosion. These risks are outweighed by long-term functional benefits.

POSTOPERATIVE CARE

After surgery, patients should refrain from lifting heavy objects and sexual activity for around six weeks. For postmenopausal women, applying local estrogen cream can enhance healing of the vaginal cuff and encourage healthy tissue regrowth. Beginning gentle pelvic-floor exercises soon after recovery and managing bowel habits to prevent constipation can further help in minimizing the chance of recurrence.

TRAINING AND FUTURE DIRECTIONS

Effective vault suspension requires thorough knowledge of pelvic anatomy along with refined laparoscopic suturing ability. Training through simulation or cadaver-based workshops helps surgeons develop these skills safely and efficiently.

Incorporating apical suspension as a standard component of total laparoscopic hysterectomy, and recording it consistently in operative reports, may enhance long-term pelvic-floor outcomes across institutions.

CONCLUSION

Restoring support at the vaginal apex is a key component of total laparoscopic hysterectomy. Among available methods, laparoscopic uterosacral ligament suspension, and McCall's Culdoplasty are supported by strong evidence for their effectiveness and low complication rates. Consistent attention to precise technique, careful protection of the ureters, and adequate surgical training can help ensure lasting prevention of vault prolapse and maintain normal vaginal structure and function.

KEY POINTS

- Restoring support at the vaginal apex is a key component of total laparoscopic hysterectomy.
- Effective vault suspension requires thorough knowledge of pelvic anatomy along with refined laparoscopic suturing ability.
- Among available methods, laparoscopic uterosacral ligament suspension, and McCall's Culdoplasty are supported by strong evidence for their effectiveness and low complication rates.
- Consistent attention to precise technique, careful protection of the ureters, and adequate surgical training can help ensure lasting prevention of vault prolapse and maintain normal vaginal structure and function.

- Training through simulation or cadaver-based workshops helps surgeons develop these skills safely and efficiently.
- Incorporating apical suspension as a standard component of total laparoscopic hysterectomy, and recording it consistently in operative reports, may enhance long-term pelvic-floor outcomes across institutions

SUGGESTED READING

1. Barber MD, Maher C. Epidemiology and outcome assessment of pelvic organ prolapse. Int Urogynecol J. 2013;24(11):1815-33.
2. Ceccaroni M, Berretta R, Malzoni M, Clarizia R, D'Agostino A, Minelli L. Laparoscopic high uterosacral ligament suspension during total laparoscopic hysterectomy: technique and outcomes. J Minim Invasive Gynecol. 2014;21(3):477-85.
3. Cruikshank SH, Kovac SR. Am J Obstet Gynecol. 1987;156:772-7.
4. DeLancey JO. Anatomic aspects of vaginal eversion after hysterectomy. Am J Obstet Gynecol. 1992;166:1717-24.
5. DeLancey JO. Anatomic aspects of vaginal eversion after hysterectomy. Am J Obstet Gynecol. 1992;167(5):1667-75.
6. Dietz HP, Simpson JM. Levator trauma is associated with pelvic organ prolapse. BJOG. 2008;115(8):979-84.
7. Haylen BT, Maher CF, Barber MD, Camargo S, Dandolu V, Digesu A, et al. An International Urogynecological Association (IUGA)/International Continence Society (ICS) joint report on the terminology for female pelvic organ prolapse (POP). Int Urogynecol J. 2016;27(4):655-84.
8. Hendrix SL, Clark A, Nygaard I, Aragaki A, Barnabei V, McTiernan A. Pelvic organ prolapse in the Women's Health Initiative: gravity and gravidity. Obstet Gynecol. 2002;100(5):981-6.
9. Jelovsek JE, Maher C, Barber MD. Pelvic organ prolapse. Lancet. 2007;369: 1027-38.
10. Kho RM, Akl MN, Cornella JL, Magtibay PM, Wechter ME, Magrina JF. Incidence and characteristics of patients with vaginal cuff dehiscence after robotic procedures. Obstet Gynecol. 2009;114(2 Pt 1):231-5.
11. Kobashi KC, Albo ME, Dmochowski RR, Ginsberg DA, Goldman HB, Gomelsky A, et al. Surgical treatment of female pelvic organ prolapse: AUA/SUFU guideline. J Urol. 2017;197(3 Pt 1):745-58.
12. Madhuri TK, Bhal K, Cross P, Odejinmi F. Laparoscopic high uterosacral ligament suspension at total laparoscopic hysterectomy for prevention of post-hysterectomy vault prolapse. J Obstet Gynaecol. 2017;37(5): 648-53.
13. Maher C, Feiner B, Baessler K, Christmann-Schmid C, Haya N, Brown J. Surgical management of pelvic organ prolapse in women. Cochrane Database Syst Rev. 2013;(4):CD004014.
14. Maher C, Feiner B, Baessler K, Christmann-Schmid C, Haya N, Brown J. Surgical management of pelvic organ prolapse in women. Cochrane Database Syst Rev. 2016;(10):CD004014.
15. Maher PJ, Chin H, Athanasiou S, Maher C. Laparoscopic management of vaginal vault prolapse: surgical techniques and outcomes. J Minim Invasive Gynecol. 2021;28(1):186-98.

16. McCall ML. Posterior culdeplasty; surgical correction of enterocele during vaginal hysterectomy; a preliminary report. Obstet Gynecol. 1957;10(6):595-602.
17. Olsen AL, Smith VJ, Bergstrom JO, Colling JC, Clark AL. Epidemiology of surgically managed pelvic organ prolapse and urinary incontinence. Obstet Gynecol. 1997;89(4):501-6.
18. Panico G, Campagna G, Caramazza D, Amato N, Ercoli A, Scambia G, et al. Laparoscopic high uterosacral ligament suspension: an alternative route for a traditional technique. Int Urogynecol J. 2018;29(8):1227-9.
19. Paul PG, Pillai R. Vault suspension at total laparoscopic hysterectomy: a new technique. Obstet Gynecol Int J. 2015;3(4):147-52.
20. Ramanah R, Berger MB, Jacquetin B, De Tayrac R. Laparoscopic uterosacral ligament suspension for apical vaginal prolapse: long-term functional and anatomical outcomes. Int Urogynecol J. 2018;29(4):585-92.
21. Rao MN, Agrawal S, Bhalerao A. Laparoscopic uterosacral plication for vault suspension during total laparoscopic hysterectomy: technique and short-term outcomes. J Gynecol Endosc Surg. 2010;2(1):25-30.
22. RCOG, BSUG. (2015) Post-Hysterectomy Vaginal Vault Prolapse. Green-top Guideline 46. [online] Available from https://www.rcog.org.uk/media/ojlovp5w/gtg-46.pdf. [Last accessed January, 2026].
23. Robinson D, et al. Int Urogynecol J. 2018;29:1-12.
24. Shull BL. Pelvic organ prolapse: anterior, superior, and posterior vaginal segment defects. Am J Obstet Gynecol. 1999;181(1):6-11.
25. Uccella S, Ceccaroni M, Alessandri F, Rosati M. Laparoscopic versus open hysterectomy for benign disease: a prospective multicenter study. Am J Obstet Gynecol. 2011;205(5):453.e1-8.
26. Vacca L, Maruccia S, Ertan K, Scioscia M, Greco P. Laparoscopic high uterosacral ligament suspension for apical support: surgical technique and medium-term outcomes. J Minim Invasive Gynecol. 2020;27(4):835-42.
27. Walters MD, Ridgeway BM. Surgical treatment of vaginal apex prolapse. Obstet Gynecol. 2013;121(2 Pt 1):354-74.

7 CHAPTER

Steps to Prevent Secondary Hemorrhage After Total Laparoscopic Hysterectomy

PG Paul

INTRODUCTION

Secondary hemorrhage occurring between 24 hours and 6 weeks after hysterectomy is a rare but life-threatening complication that may require prompt medical and surgical intervention. Although the overall incidence of secondary hemorrhage is low, gynecologists do encounter cases of varying severity. Though the reported incidence ranges between 0.9 and 1.5%, recent evidence suggests it may be more frequent after TLH compared to abdominal or vaginal routes. This trend likely reflects the widespread adoption of energy-based dissection techniques that, while effective for hemostasis, can produce localized tissue necrosis and delayed sloughing. The condition is clinically significant as patients often present with profuse vaginal bleeding, necessitating emergency management. A clear understanding of causative mechanisms and preventive strategies is therefore vital for all laparoscopic surgeons. A few publications are available on secondary hemorrhage following hysterectomy. So this chapter is mainly based on my two publications on secondary hemorrhage— one after TLH and the other, a comparison of the three types of hysterectomy.

PATHOPHYSIOLOGY OF SECONDARY HEMORRHAGE

The pathogenesis of secondary hemorrhage is primarily related to delayed disruption of small vessels within the healing vaginal vault or paracervical tissues. During TLH, the uterine arteries and vaginal cuff are sealed using bipolar or ultrasonic energy. This creates a zone of coagulative necrosis extending 1–2 mm beyond the coagulated area. Over the subsequent days, inflammatory infiltration and tissue liquefaction lead to the separation of the eschar and the reopening of sealed vessels. This usually occurs between 10 and 14 days postoperatively—the period of granulation and epithelial regeneration.

Large uteri and extensive dissection increase tissue devascularization, while infection or hematoma delays re-epithelialization, predisposing to vessel exposure and secondary bleeding. Overuse of thermal energy can cause deeper necrosis and delayed sloughing. Premature resumption of intercourse or heavy physical activity may mechanically disrupt the fragile healing cuff. The usual bleeding source is the vault itself, although rare cases of pseudoaneurysm of the uterine or vaginal artery have been described.

PREOPERATIVE CONSIDERATIONS

Prevention begins with careful patient optimization before surgery. Correction of anemia and coagulopathy is essential to reduce perioperative and postoperative risk. Active vaginal or cervical infections should be treated preoperatively, as infection is strongly associated with cuff dehiscence and delayed bleeding. Detailed imaging evaluation of uterine size and pathology guides surgical planning—uteri weighing over 500 g pose a higher risk of postoperative bleeding owing to increased vascularity and traction on pedicles.

Preoperative counseling should stress postoperative restrictions and early reporting of any bleeding. Prophylactic antibiotics are administered at induction and repeated once postoperatively. Surgeons must ensure familiarity with the specific energy source being used, as variations in power output, waveform, and thermal spread can influence tissue necrosis and healing.

INTRAOPERATIVE PREVENTIVE STEPS

The intraoperative phase offers the most incredible opportunity to prevent secondary hemorrhage. The uterine arteries should be skeletonized before sealing, allowing efficient energy delivery at the vessel wall while sparing adjacent tissues. Bipolar coagulation should continue only until blanching occurs; excessive energy application or charring predisposes to deep necrosis.

During colpotomy, a pure-cut monopolar current (60 W) is preferred to minimize lateral heat spread. The incision should be placed slightly above the uterosacral attachments to preserve the vascular arcade that supports the vaginal cuff. In postmenopausal or atrophic tissues, minimal thermal energy should be used.

After specimen removal, meticulous inspection of the vaginal cuff is mandatory. The field should be irrigated and dried; even minor oozing must be controlled. Full-thickness vault closure with delayed absorbable suture is recommended. The sutures should include the uterosacral ligaments at the angles to maintain vascularity and cuff support. Each suture bite should include 1 cm of tissue to prevent ischemic margins. Few reports suggest the use of an additional reinforcing layer of sutures, mainly to avoid vault dehiscence. We always use a single layer of sutures. We now prefer barbed sutures for all laparoscopic vault closure.

Vault sealing with excessive bipolar energy or overuse of ultrasonic shears must be avoided. When available, power settings should be adjusted to achieve effective hemostasis without carbonization. Instruments should be cleaned periodically during surgery to prevent arcing. The final inspection should ensure that the vault is dry and clean before closure.

POSTOPERATIVE MEASURES

Immediate postoperative vigilance is critical. Patients with persistent tachycardia or vaginal bleeding warrant prompt examination. Early ambulation is encouraged, but strenuous exercise, squatting, or lifting weights must be avoided for at least 6 weeks. Intercourse should be deferred until 6-8 weeks post-surgery.

Signs of infection, such as fever, pelvic pain, or discharge between days 7 and 14, require evaluation. Ultrasonography may reveal a vault hematoma, which can serve as a nidus for infection and delayed bleeding. Antibiotic coverage should include anaerobic organisms. Prompt treatment prevents progression to secondary hemorrhage.

MANAGEMENT OF SECONDARY HEMORRHAGE

Although preventive measures minimize the risk, occasional cases still occur. Management requires a structured approach. The priority is hemodynamic stabilization with intravenous fluids and, if necessary, cross-matched blood. Examination under anesthesia helps identify the bleeding site. In most cases, tight vaginal packing with sterile gauze controls bleeding within hours. If oozing persists, resuturing of the vault edges with delayed-absorbable material is indicated. Necrotic or infected tissue should be debrided gently to expose viable bleeding edges.

If bleeding in the pelvic cavity is identified, diagnostic laparoscopy may be undertaken to inspect the vault, uterine pedicles, and adjacent structures. Laparoscopic bipolar coagulation of the uterine artery may be performed when active bleeding is visualized. This approach avoids the morbidity of laparotomy. We had performed laparoscopy only once in our series. In patients with recurrent bleeding, selective uterine or vaginal artery embolization by interventional radiology is now the treatment of choice, providing effective and minimally invasive control. Rarely, pseudoaneurysms have been identified as the source, emphasizing the need for imaging when bleeding persists after initial control.

CONCLUSION

Secondary hemorrhage following TLH, though rare, demands serious attention because of its unpredictable onset and potential severity. The most important preventive strategy is meticulous surgical technique: precise energy application, adequate hemostasis, and sound vault closure. Large uteri, excessive energy use, and postoperative infection remain consistent risk factors. A proactive approach—emphasizing preoperative optimization, intraoperative precision, and patient education—can minimize risk.

Surgeons must also recognize the importance of training and standardization. Early in the learning curve, overuse of energy devices and inadequate vault suturing contribute disproportionately to complications. Adherence to established energy settings, magnified visualization, and a dry operative field are essential habits. Ultimately, prevention depends on three principles: a dry vault at the end of surgery, a clean vault during recovery, and an informed patient who seeks help early. Adopting these measures ensures safer outcomes in laparoscopic hysterectomy.

KEY POINTS

Secondary hemorrhage after total laparoscopic hysterectomy (TLH) is an uncommon but serious complication occurring 1–6 weeks post-surgery, mainly due to thermal necrosis, infection, or inadequate vault healing. The risk is higher with large uteri, excessive energy use, or vault infection. Prevention requires meticulous surgical technique—skeletonizing uterine arteries before sealing, using controlled energy for colpotomy, ensuring full-thickness vault closure with uterosacral support, and confirming a dry field before closure. Strict asepsis, antibiotic cover, and avoidance of premature physical activity further reduce risk. Postoperative vigilance for pain, fever, or spotting enables early detection of infection or hematoma. When secondary bleeding occurs, vaginal packing controls most cases; persistent bleeding may require vault resuturing, laparoscopic hemostasis, or uterine artery embolization. A dry vault at surgery, a clean vault during recovery, and an informed patient form the triad of prevention, ensuring safer outcomes after TLH.

SUGGESTED READING

1. Holub Z, Jabor A. Laparoscopic management of bleeding after laparoscopic or vaginal hysterectomy. JSLS. 2004;8:235-8.
2. Paul PG, Panditrao AS, Khan S, Talwar P, Kaur H, Barsagade S. Secondary hemorrhage after different modes of hysterectomy. Gynecol Surg. 2013;10:267-72.
3. Paul PG, Talwar P, Kaur H, Shabnam K, Kandhari D, Chopade G. Secondary Hemorrhage After Total Laparoscopic Hysterectomy. JSLS. 2014;18(3):e2014.00139.
4. Pragash V, Reddy SD. Secondary Hemorrhage After Total Laparoscopic Hysterectomy: An Observational Study. Cureus. 2025;17(3):e79956.
5. Takeda A, Koyama K, Mori M, Sakai K, Mitsui T, Nakamura H. Diagnostic CT angiography and embolization for postoperative hemorrhage after gynecologic laparoscopy. J Minim Invasive Gynecol. 2008;15:332-41.

8 CHAPTER

Complications of Laparoscopy

Nikita Trehan, Subash Mallya, Divya TN, Ritu Jain

INTRODUCTION

Minimally invasive gynecologic surgery offers superior cosmetic results, shorter recovery, reduced postoperative pain, and shorter hospital stays. Yet, they carry inherent risks. Complications may arise intraoperatively or postoperatively, ranging from minor injuries to life-threatening events **(Box 1)**. In recent

BOX 1: Types of laparoscopic complications.

Injuries to intra-abdominal structures:
- Bowel wall or solid organ injuries (e.g., perforation, contusion)
- Bladder/Ureteral or other retroperitoneal structure injury
- Vascular injuries (e.g., vessel laceration, bleeding)
- Nerve injuries (e.g., omental, or mesenteric vessels with traction)

Anesthesia-related complications:
- Difficult airway and ventilation issues
- Reactions to anesthesia agents (hypotension, bradycardia, tachycardia, malignant hyperthermia in susceptible individuals)
- Aspiration risk or airway edema
- Depth/monitoring-related complications (inadequate depth, hemodynamic instability)

Pneumoperitoneum-related complications:
- Cardiovascular: Decreased venous return, arrhythmias, hypotension
- Respiratory: Reduced lung compliance, hypercarbia, hypoxemia
- Gas embolism (rare)
- Subcutaneous emphysema or pneumothorax
- Shoulder tip pain due to diaphragmatic irritation

Procedure-specific complications (e.g., mesh usage):
- Mesh-related: Infection, adhesion formation, mesh migration, or erosion
- Parasitic Fibroids: Small Fibroid tissues inadvertently left behind.
- Inadequate tissue approximation: Intramyometrial abscess, Scar Implantation- Post-Myomectomy
- Complications from improper closure of fascial defects (port-site hernias)

Other technical or iatrogenic issues:
- Poor visualization leading to misidentification of structures
- Thermal/energy device injuries to vessels, nerves, or organs
- Instrument breakage or unintended tissue traction
- Port-site complications (Seroma, Hematoma, Hernia, etc.

years, rapid expansion of Endoscopy has shown parallel rise in complications affecting multiple organ systems.

Comprehensive precautions, meticulous technique, and prompt management are essential to minimize morbidity.

ENTRY-RELATED COMPLICATIONS

>50% Laparoscopy-related complications occur during entry, with injuries most often involving vascular, urinary, or gastrointestinal structures. Cochrane Database reported bowel injury ~1.8, vascular injury ~0.9, extraperitoneal insufflation or failed entry, at ~20 per 1,000.

Three primary entry techniques are widely used, each with distinct advantages: Veress needle with prior CO_2 insufflation, Direct trocar insertion and Open (Hasson) approach.

Crucial steps to minimize injury include elevating abdominal wall by manual lifting, elevating umbilical edges with clamps, or lateral elevation of wall using clamps. If two Veress needle attempts fail, alternative entry methods are recommended.

In selecting a primary entry site, patient history is important. In patients with previous midline laparotomy, it is advisable to avoid umbilicus and consider Palmer's or Lee-Huang's point for safer entry. The Jain point has emerged as a newer non-umbilical access site. Alternate entry points through the cul-de-sac **(Fig. 1)** or transuterine approaches suggested. A nasogastric tube may be employed to mitigate stomach injury when high-entry points are used.

Affected structures: Small intestine (25%), Iliac artery (19%), Colon (12%), iliac and other retroperitoneal veins (9%), mesenteric artery (7%), aorta (6%), inferior vena cava (4%), abdominal wall vessels (4%), bladder (3%), and liver (2%).

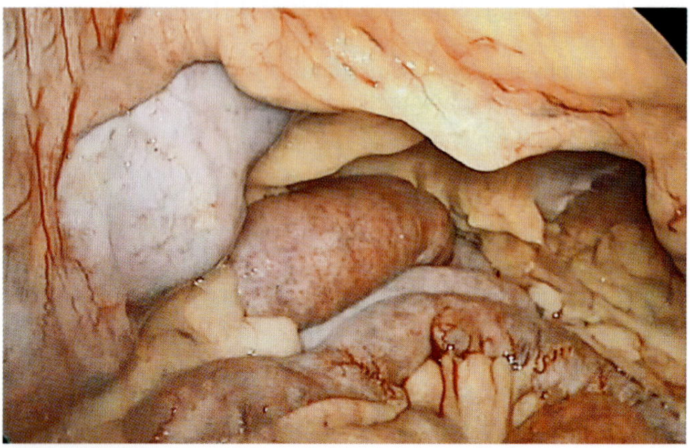

Fig. 1: Entry thru the cul de sac in a case of previous splenectomy.

BOWEL INJURIES (TABLE 1)

Injury to the small bowel and rectosigmoid colon is common during entry or improper use of thermal energy. These injuries may go unnoticed intraoperatively, leading to delayed diagnosis, peritonitis, severe intra-abdominal infections, and sepsis. Delayed recognition being leading cause of laparoscopy-related mortality.

In prior mesh repair, bowel can adhere to mesh; thus, entry should be marked 2 cm away and lateral from prior mesh sites. In cases of trocar bowel entry, trocar should not be withdrawn; instead, an alternative entry site used to avoid losing the injured area. Post-adhesiolysis, meticulous exploration is necessary to identify additional injuries ("through-and-through" injuries/ entry and exit). Bowel injury during Adhesiolysis, in prior surgery, infection, or endometriosis cases is possible; repair is typically performed in two layers **(Fig. 2)**. Safety leak tests with methylene blue or air/water immersion should be conducted **(Figs. 3A and B)**. An omental patch may be applied to reinforce repair. Primary repair is feasible in most cases; covering stoma may be required if late presentation with peritonitis has occurred. Following injury repair, a large-bore drain (e.g., 32 Fr chest tube drain) and broad-spectrum antibiotics are recommended. Rarely, bowel injury may be complicated by inadvertent morcellation during fibroid morcellation **(Fig. 4)**.

TABLE 1: Adhesion and bowel injury risk according to route of surgery.

	Adhesions (risk in %)	*Bowel injury (risk in %)*
No surgery	0.68%	0.42%
Laparoscopy	1.6%	0.8%
Pfannsteil	19.8%	6.4%
Midline incision	57.1%	31.8%

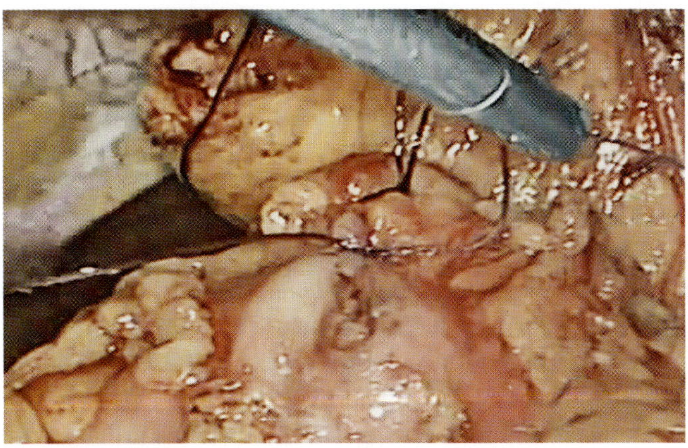

Fig. 2: The bowel is sutured in two layers using 2-0 vicryl/pds.

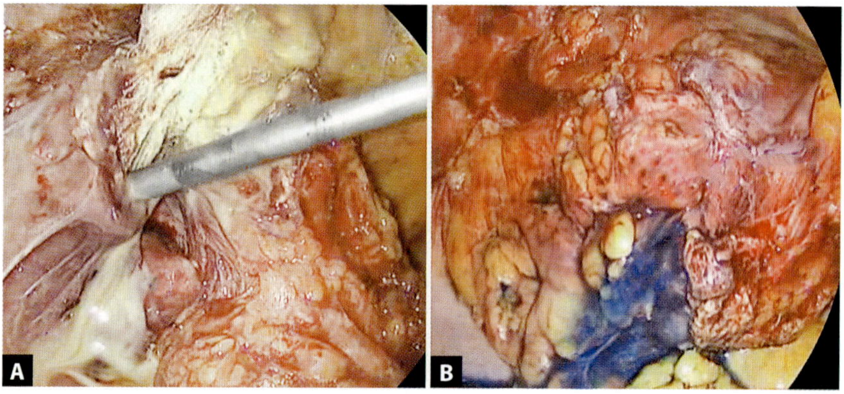

Figs. 3A and B: A rare case of Gossypiboma where a gauze piece was left during a previous laparotomy the sigmoid colon was injured during Adhesiolysis and the injury was identified during a methylene blue leak test. The rent was repaired in 2 layers.

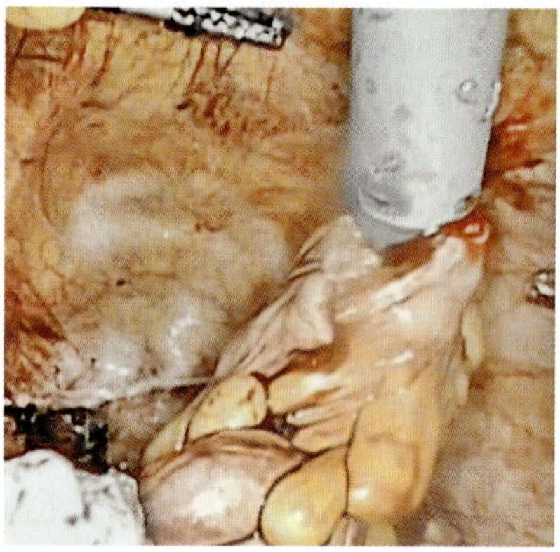

Fig. 4: Inadvertent bowel morcellation.
Source: Internet.

BLADDER INJURIES

Bladder injuries are more common in laparoscopy than ureteric injuries and are typically identified earlier. Risk factors include prior pelvic surgery, infection, endometriosis, pelvic tumors, and other conditions that distort pelvic anatomy. Mechanisms include thermal injury, transection, ligation, retraction, contusion, or devascularization, and injuries may be unrecognized during surgery. Approximately 90% of bladder injuries are detected intraoperatively, and associated morbidity is generally low. Common scenarios for bladder injury include: Suprapubic trocar insertion, Adherent Bladder dissection in prior surgical cases, Dissection in vault surgeries **(Fig. 5)**, Excessive use of thermal energy.

Intraoperative recognition is suggested by observed urinary leakage or air in urobag. Bladder endometriosis may necessitate partial or full-thickness

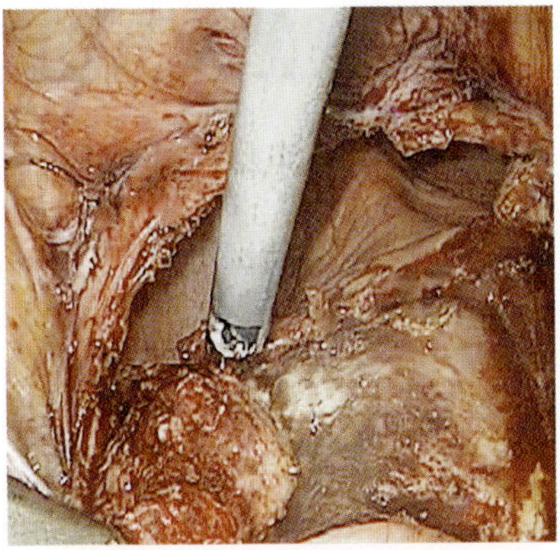

Fig. 5: Bladder injury during bladder separation from vault in vault prolapse.

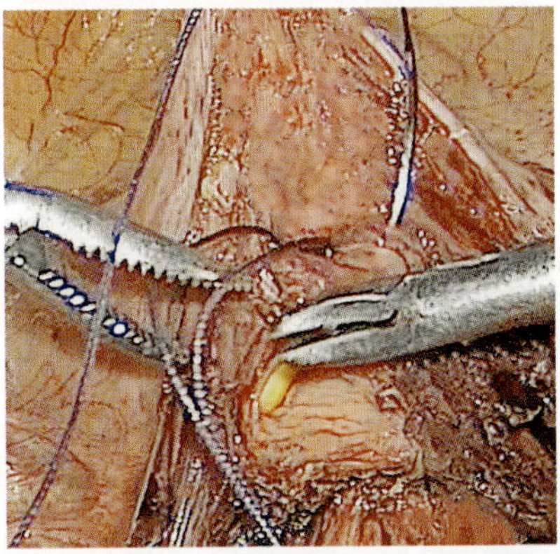

Fig. 6: A full thickness bladder cystectomy being carried out for a bladder endometriotic nodule. Bladder being stitched with vicryl sutures.

resection in cases of endometriotic nodules. Supra Trigonal Repairs are typically performed with absorbable sutures (3-0 Vicryl or PDS) in two layers **(Fig. 6)**; barbed sutures are also an option. If injury is near ureteric orifices, pre-repair ureteric catheterization or stenting is advised. A Foley catheter is typically left in place for about 10 days to ensure bladder drainage. In cases of thermal injury with necrosis, resection of the necrotic area precedes repair. Concurrent injuries to posterior bladder and vagina may result in vesicovaginal or ureterovaginal fistula, which should be repaired with an omental patch between suture lines if needed.

URETERIC INJURIES

Ureteral injuries occur even during seemingly straightforward procedures (e.g., TLH) and are more likely with expanded dissection in extra pelvic endometriosis, large ovarian masses, cervical/broad ligament fibroids, or extensive pelvic adhesions. Ureterolysis should be performed as needed.

Mechanisms of ureteral injury include: Laceration during sharp dissection, Devascularization from adventitial damage, kinking (Mac Calls Culdoplasty or Moscowitz Procedure), Thermal injury from lateral spread of bipolar or monopolar energy, Transection, or overzealous use of ultrasonic devices.

Majority present in immediate postoperative period with flank pain, nausea, fever, and sometimes elevated creatinine, though thermal injuries can present later. Ureteral stricture may cause hydroureter, elevated creatinine, and urinoma formation, leading to severe peritoneal irritation and pain.

Ultrasound or IVP can be used, but CT urography is the investigation of choice.

Management: Cystoscopic stenting facilitates healing (6 weeks). Mid-ureteral injuries require end-to-end anastomosis (+/– proximal spatulation) **(Fig. 7)**. Distal ureteral injuries are managed with ureteroneocystostomy; if tension anticipated, psoas-hitch procedure reduces distortion and tension **(Fig. 8)**. Ureteric catheters removed after 6–8 weeks following repair.

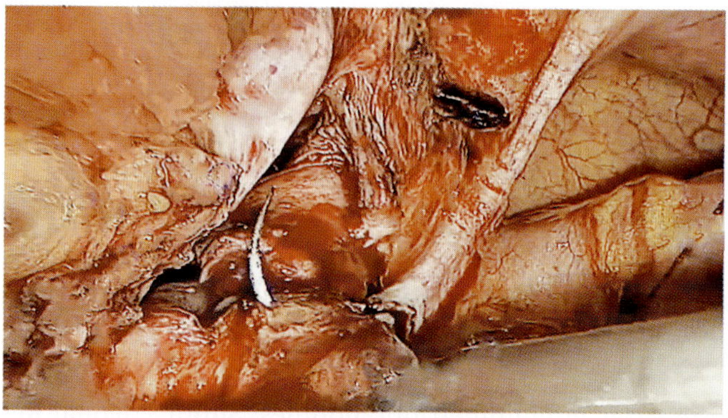

Fig. 7: End-to-end ureteric anastomosis being carried out over a stent.

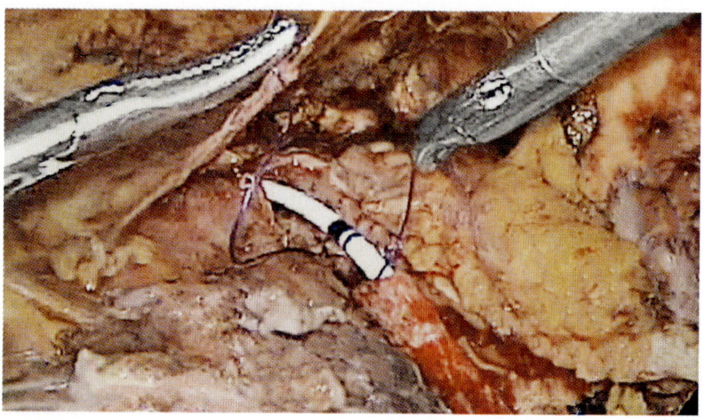

Fig. 8: Ureter being implanted into the bladder after releasing the bladder from the space of Retzius and performing a psoas hitch in a case of ureteric endometriosis.

VASCULAR INJURIES

Majority vascular injury occurs at Veress needle or primary trocar insertion but also during lymphadenectomy and potentially from active electrocautery or laser overshoot.

Key preventive measures include:

- Understand anatomy: Aortic bifurcation lies around L4, with retroperitoneal vessels 2–5 cm from umbilicus; lifting abdominal wall with one hand remains important across all patients.
- Entry technique: Use uniform, steady trocar insertion with controlled force; avoid excessive force, especially with small skin incisions **(Fig. 9)**
- Adequate incision size: Sufficiently large primary trocar incision to reduce need for forceful entry and trocar overshoot.
- Positioning: Avoid Trendelenburg for primary trocar entry.
- Preparedness: Keeping Vascular clamps and laparotomy trolley ready in OR is advisable **(Figs. 10A to G)**.
- Retroperitoneal dissection strategy: Open peritoneum widely and develop avascular spaces to anticipate and control potential vascular or nerve injuries laparoscopically.
- During paraaortic lymphadenectomy, arterial injuries may occur, sometimes requiring arteriorrhaphy or repair with monofilament sutures. If stenosis risk is high or repair is unlikely to maintain lumen integrity, patch angioplasty or grafting may be indicated.
- Venous injuries to common iliac vein or, rarely, inferior vena cava, can be sutured laparoscopically with 6-0 monofilament sutures after gentle retraction of vein edges.
- Venous bleeding from deeply situated sacral vessels during Sacro colpopexy, vessels in corona mortis during Paravesical space dissection,

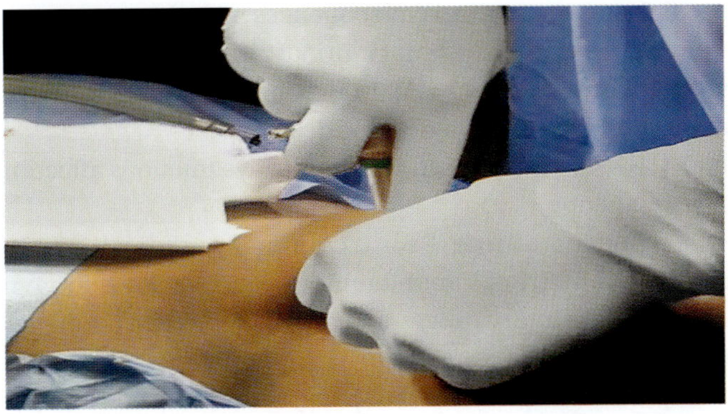

Fig. 9: The surgeon lifts the anterior abdominal wall with her left hand and inserts the trocar steadily with her right hand while using the index finger of her right hand as a guard to prevent overshooting.

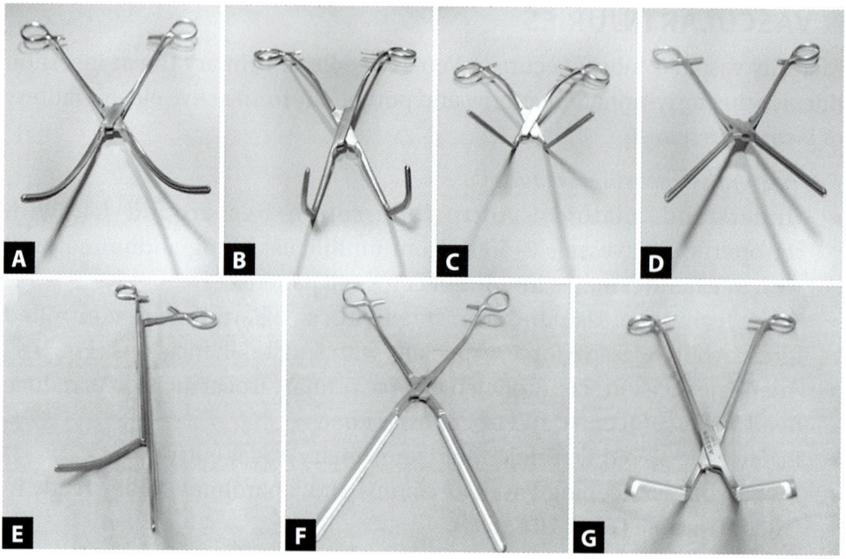

Figs. 10A to G: (A) DeBakey; (B) Satinsky; (C) Femoral; (D) Iliac; (E) Chitwood; (F) Straight handle Fogarty; and (G) Angled handle Fogarty.

or circle of death during inguinal hernia repair can be particularly challenging to manage.

- Involvement of vascular surgeons and postoperative ICU care are essential to reduce morbidity; postoperative anticoagulation is typically continued for about 6 months.

NERVE INJURIES

The pelvic autonomic nervous system comprises sympathetic components (superior hypogastric plexus and hypogastric nerves) and parasympathetic components (pelvic splanchnic nerves) and Inferior hypogastric plexus (IHP). Specific neuroanatomical consequences include:

- Superior hypogastric plexus injury: urinary urgency or incontinence.
- Pelvic splanchnic nerve or IHP injury: bladder atony, altered bladder sensation, and decreased vaginal lubrication.
- IHP injury: Spectrum of mixed autonomic dysfunctions affecting urinary and sexual function.

Injury can occur during Sacro colpopexy, radical hysterectomy, rectovaginal endometriosis management, and various urogynecology procedures. Avoiding injury hinges on employing nerve-sparing techniques and limiting dissection within high-risk planes. For example, limiting dissection in pararectal space (Latzko space) above deep uterine vein reduces pelvic splanchnic nerve injury risk. When dissecting near the bladder, attention to bladder pillars and maintaining medial-to-ureter dissection (Yabuki's space) helps preserve autonomic innervation.

Somatic nerves: Genitofemoral nerve injury can result in sensory loss over anterior medial thigh, whereas obturator nerve injury during pelvic lymphadenectomy can cause dysesthesia, adduction weakness, and adductor muscle atrophy. Nerve injury may require repair with nonabsorbable sutures such as 6-0 Prolene.

MESH-RELATED (PROLAPSE SURGERY)

Mesh use necessitates meticulous patient optimization and adherence to best practices to minimize complications:

- *Preoperative optimization:* Address obesity, smoking, and diabetes to reduce morbidity.
- *Mesh selection and infection risk:* prefer monofilament macroporous meshes (>75 μm pore size) to facilitate immune clearance; avoid mesh placement after rectal repair due to infection and erosion risk.
- *Hemostasis:* Ensure perfect hemostasis to prevent hematoma-related infection.
- *Mesh exposure and vault considerations:* Limit mesh exposure to vagina; consider subtotal hysterectomy to reduce exposure risk; perform mesh peritonealization to prevent bowel entrapment.
- *Over-tension and dissection:* Use wide, loose mesh to avoid dyspareunia and chronic pain; avoid overtightening and ensure adequate space for tissue dynamics.

PORT SITE HERNIA

Postoperative hernia risk after laparoscopy is markedly lower than abdominal surgery. Trocar-site fascial closure (>5 mm Ports) reduces port-site hernias; bladeless trocars further lower risk. Open Fascia closure technique or port closure devices (Carter–Thomason/Endo close, etc.) can be used.

UNIQUE COMPLICATIONS

- *Parasitic fibroids:* Morcellation can disseminate fragments, leading to parasitic fibroids supplied by omental, mesenteric, or hepatic vasculature; Endo bag morcellation mitigates this risk **(Fig. 11)**
- *Intra-myometrial abscess:* Poorly sutured myometrial beds may accumulate hematomas infected by bacteria **(Fig. 12)**.
- *Intra-myometrial pregnancy:* Scar ectopic after myomectomy requires prudent devascularization prior to evacuation and layered closure of myometrium to prevent hematoma and weak scarring.

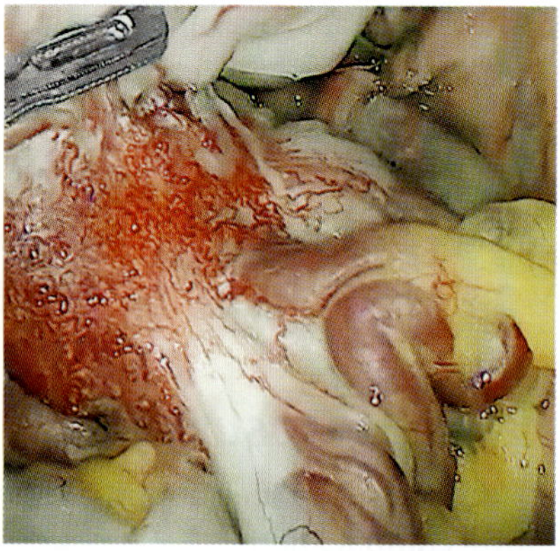

Fig. 11: A large parasitic fibroid attached to the bowel.

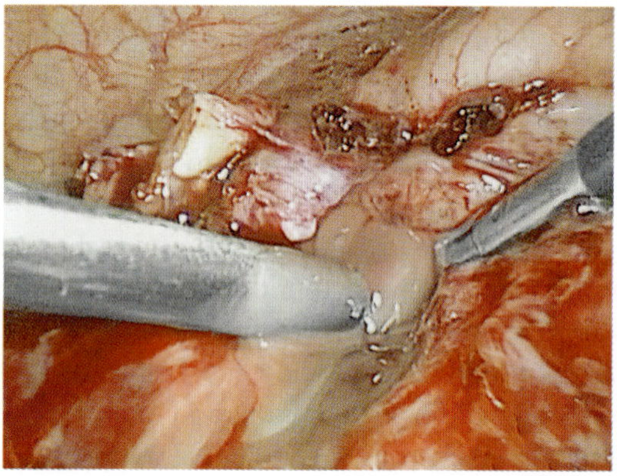

Fig. 12: Pelvic abscess in a myoma bed being drained after separating bowel adhesions.

KEY POINTS

- Entry complications are most common and include bowel, vascular, and urinary tract injuries. Careful planning of entry technique and entry-site selection, particularly in patients with prior abdominal surgeries or mesh repairs, can mitigate risk.
- *Safe entry techniques:* Closed (Veress), Open (Hasson) and Direct. Stop after two failed Veress attempts and shift to alternative entry methods.
- Palmer's point, Lee Huang's and Jain's point can be used as alternative port sites in previously operated abdomen.
- Secondary ports must be inserted under direct vision.
- Maintain low intraperitoneal pressure and free gas flow for safe access.
- *Recommended insufflation pressures:* 20–25 mm Hg during entry, reduce to 12–15 mm Hg for surgery.
- Thermal injuries possible with energy devices—use with caution.
- Early recognition of injuries reduces morbidity.

- Bowel injuries carry significant morbidity and mortality when undetected; meticulous intraoperative assessment and prompt repair are essential.
- Bladder injuries, though often identified intraoperatively, require prompt repair and postoperative catheter drainage to ensure healing and prevent fistula formation.
- Ureteric injuries require high clinical vigilance, especially in high-risk scenarios. Timely imaging (CT urography) and urologic repair (stenting, ureteral reconstruction) are critical for favorable outcomes.
- Vascular, Nerve, and Visceral injuries are recognized risks of laparoscopic surgery.
- Retroperitoneal vascular injuries can occur at entry (Veress needle or primary trocar) and may arise later during lymphadenectomy or from unintended energy device effects.
- Overall, minimizing complications hinges on careful technique, thorough acknowledgment of patient's history, vigilant intraoperative assessment, and prompt diagnostic and therapeutic interventions when injuries are identified.
- Adequate training, simulation practice, and familiarity with equipment are critical.

SUGGESTED READING

1. Berker B, Taskın S, Taskın E. Complications of Laparoscopic Gynecologic Surgery. In: Michael S (Ed). Prevention and Management of Laparoendoscopic Surgical Complications, 3rd edition. USA: Society of Laparoendoscopic Surgeons; 2012.
2. Crist DW, Gadacz TR. Complications of laparoscopic surgery. Surg Clin North Am. 1993;73(2):265-89.
3. Härkki-Siren P, Sjoberg J, Kurki T. Major complications of laparoscopy: A follow-up Finnish study. Obstet Gynecol. 1999;94(1):94-8.
4. Jain N, Jain V, Chandi A, Srivastava S, Singh S, Vasundhara N. Jain point: an alternate laparoscopic non-umbilical first blind entry port to avoid vessel, viscera, adhesions and bowel (VVAB). Updates Surg. 2021;73(6):2321-9.
5. Magrina JF. Complications of laparoscopic surgery. Clin Obstet Gynecol. 2002;45(2):469-80.
6. Peterson HB, Hulka JF, Phillips JM. American Association of Gynecologic Laparoscopists' 1988 membership survey on operative laparoscopy. J Reprod Med. 1990;35(6):587-9.
7. Roy GM, Bazzurini L, Solima E, Luciano AA. Safe technique for laparoscopic entry into the abdominal cavity. J Am Assoc Gynecol Laparosc. 2001;8(4):519-28.
8. Yuzpe AA. Pneumoperitoneum needle and trocar injuries in laparoscopy. A survey on possible contributing factors and prevention. J Reprod Med. 1990;35(5):485-90.

9 CHAPTER

Safe Abdominal Entry

Amit Tandon, Akriti Prajapati

INTRODUCTION

Abdominal access during laparoscopy is a vital step and must be performed with great precision. Although laparoscopy offers numerous advantages such as reduced postoperative morbidity, shorter hospital stay, and faster recovery, most of the serious complications occur during the initial access phase. Injury to major vessels, bowel, or bladder can result from improper entry techniques, poor visualization, or anatomical variations. Therefore, a sound understanding of the principles of abdominal access, selection of entry technique and awareness of anatomical landmarks is essential to minimize risks.

ANATOMY OF ANTERIOR ABDOMINAL WALL (FIGS. 1 TO 3)

Knowledge of the surgical anatomy of the abdominal wall is fundamental to ensuring safe laparoscopic access.

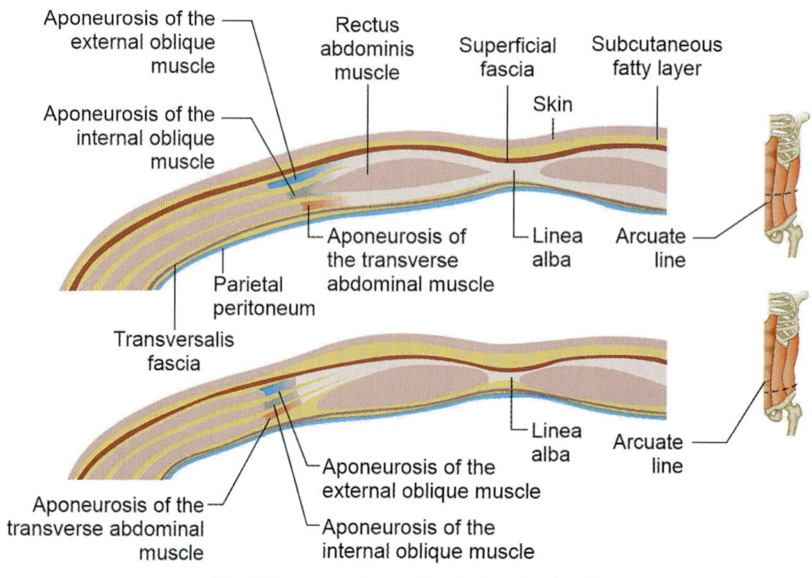

Fig. 1: Layers of anterior abdominal wall.

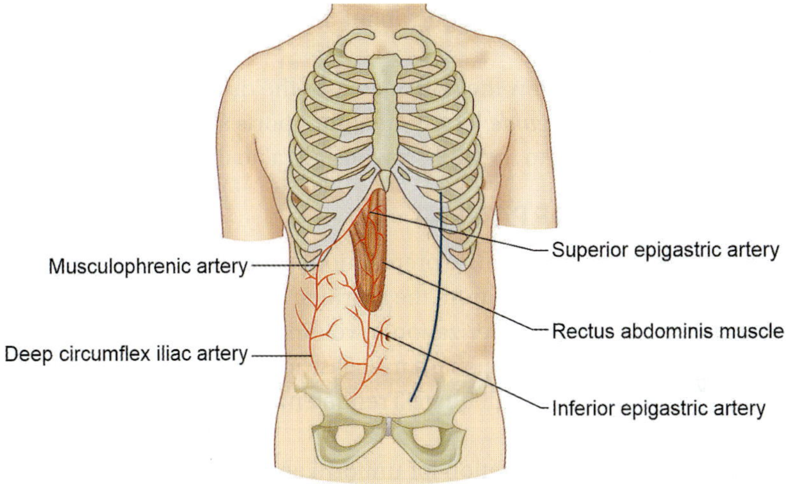

Fig. 2: Vascular supply of anterior abdominal wall.

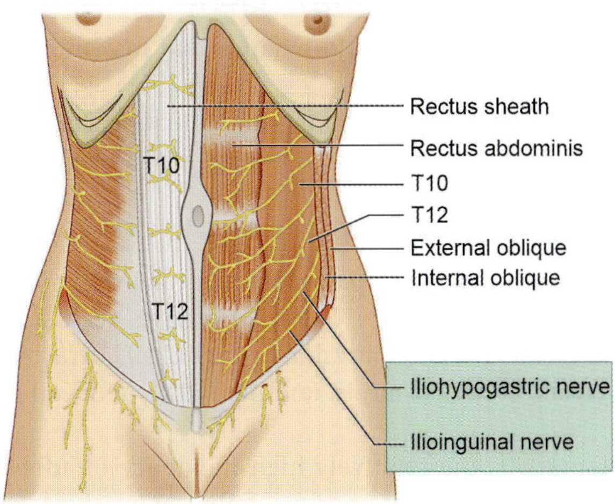

Fig. 3: Nerve Supply of Anterior Abdominal Wall.

Umbilicus

- Preferred site of access for the majority of laparoscopic procedure
- Fusion of fascial layers and peritoneum with minimal fat
- *Inferior epigastric artery:* Most important and largest blood vessel of anterior abdominal wall
- Avoid the *danger zone* between *3 and 8 cm from the midline* to prevent injury to the inferior epigastric vessels. Entry medial or lateral to this area is considered safe.
- *Ilioinguinal and iliohypogastric nerves* run along the lateral border of psoas and enter the transversus abdominis near the anterior iliac crest.

- They pierce the internal oblique about 3 cm medial and 3.5 cm inferior to the ASIS.
- Trocar placement below the ASIS increases the risk of nerve injury.
- *Safe port placement guide:* Lower quadrant ports should be placed 2 cm medial and superior to the ASIS, staying lateral to the rectus border.

PREPARATION OF PATIENT

- Ensure thorough preoperative preparation to reduce access injuries.
- Patient must be kept NPO from the morning of the scheduled surgery.
- Empty the bladder (catheterization or voiding) before entry.
- Decompress the stomach using a nasogastric tube to prevent injury.
- Position the patient in adequate Trendelenburg to elevate the anterior abdominal wall.
- Achieve full muscle relaxation for uniform abdominal wall elevation and easier trocar insertion.

SELECTING AN APPROPRIATE ENTRY SITE (TABLE 1)

The optimal entry location should balance and maximize the following factors:

- Avoidance of critical extra- and intra-abdominal structures
- Proximity to the target anatomy or underlying pathology

UMBILICAL POINT (FIG. 4)

- Preferred entry site in most laparoscopic procedures.
- Advantages: Ease of entry, better operative access to the pelvic structures, greater port mobility due to the lack of lateral resistance from adipose layers, better cosmesis, and potentially reduced postoperative pain.
- A disadvantage is the relatively high incidence of adhesions in this region among patients with previous umbilical incisions. Infraumbilical adhesions have been observed in approximately 30% to 50% of patients with a previous midline vertical incision.

LEFT UPPER QUADRANT OR PALMER'S POINT (FIG. 5)

Palmer point is located 3 cm below the left subcostal margin in the midclavicular line.

Indications:

- Infraumbilical laparotomy scar present
- Three failed trans-umbilical entry attempts
- Obese or very thin patients

Contraindications:

- Prior splenic or gastric surgery
- Hepatosplenomegaly

TABLE 1: Comparisons of different entry techniques.

Entry technique	*Advantages*	*Disadvantages*
Open (Hasson) Technique	• Avoidance of blind puncture with a Veress needle, following trocar insertion • Establishing a pneumoperitoneum • Correct anatomical repair of the abdominal wall incision • Significant reduction of failed entry as compared to closed entry technique	• Longer time consumption • Difficult technique • Pneumoperitoneum maintenance • Not suitable in Obese Patients
Closed (Veress) Needle Technique	• Limited incision site resulting in minimal tissue trauma and better cosmetic outcome • Minimal gas loss during insufflation • Widely used and well understood	• Higher incidence of failed entry • Extraperitoneal insufflation • Omental injury • Intestinal insufflation • CO_2 embolism
Optical (Direct vision) access Technique	• Early detection of injury • Direct visualization during entry	• Requires special equipment • Risk of thermal fogging or poor visualization
Direct Trocar Entry Technique	• Prevention of complications associated with Veress needle use • Faster than any other entry technique	Least performed in clinical practice today

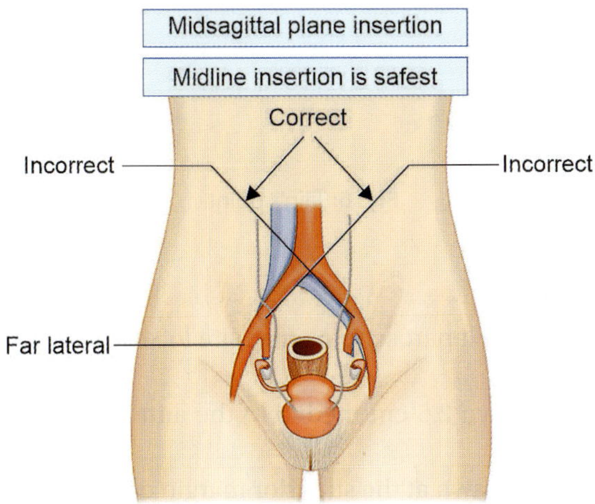

Fig. 4: Site of umbilical port placement.

- Portal hypertension
- Gastro-pancreatic masses
- Improper nasogastric tube placement causing gastric distension

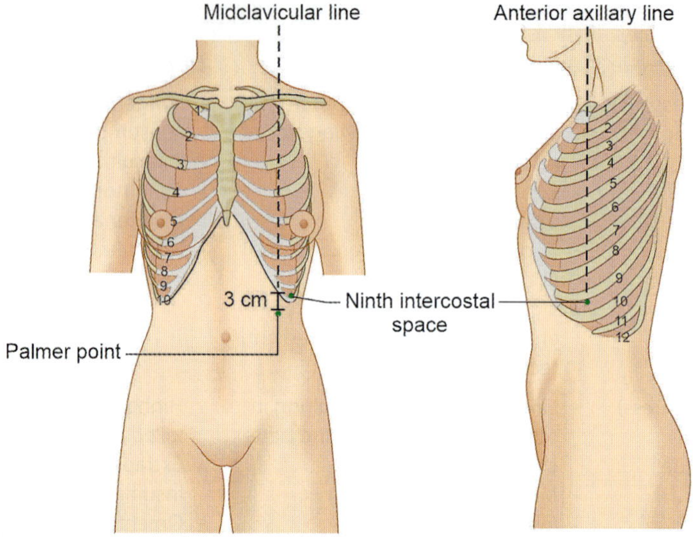

Fig. 5: Left upper quadrant or palmer's point

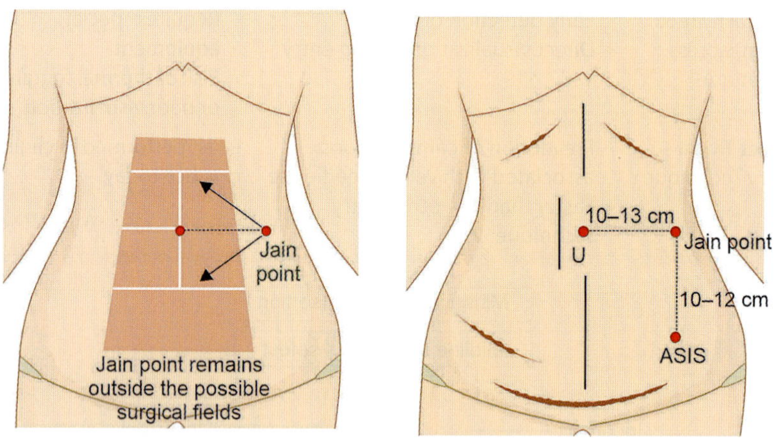

Fig. 6: Jain's point.

JAIN'S POINT

The Jain point is a safe laparoscopic entry site located at the intersection of two lines **(Fig. 6)**:

- A vertical line drawn 2.5 cm medial to the anterior superior iliac spine (ASIS)
- A horizontal line drawn at the superior margin of the umbilicus
- Learning curve is short
- Serves as the primary ergonomic working port
- No known contraindications
- Can be mirrored on the right side

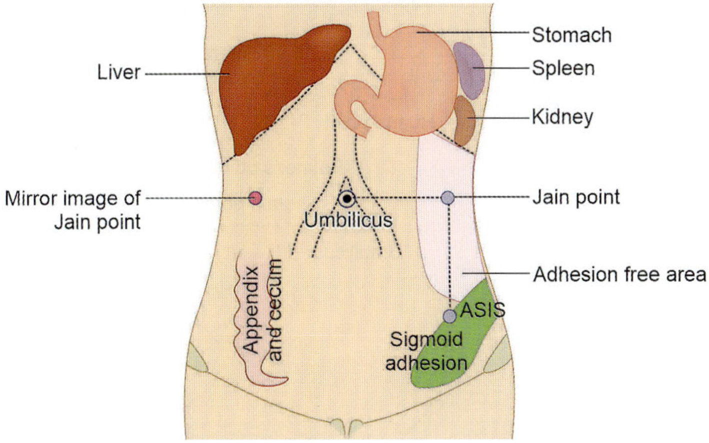

Fig. 7: Anatomical considerations of Jain's point.

- Can be used in upper abdominal scars
- Allows safe entry in cases of suspected upper abdominal adhesions

ANATOMICAL CONSIDERATIONS

The Jain point is located at the L4 level, 10–13 cm lateral to the umbilicus on the left side. It lies safely away from the viscera—including the spleen, kidney, and distended stomach—as well as the sigmoid colon, within a broad nascent area extending from L1 to the pelvis. This region is generally free of major vessels, viscera, adhesions, and bowel, making it a safe site for laparoscopic entry **(Fig. 7)**.

LEE–HUANG POINT (FIG. 8)

Lee-Huang Point is a laparoscopic entry site located midway between the xiphoid process and the umbilicus on the midline of the abdomen.

ADVANTAGES

- Central position ensures a direct, symmetrical view of the pelvis
- Offers a higher vantage point than umbilical access, it provides a broader, elevated view of the operative field without needing to reposition the telescope.

Indications:

- Large pelvic pathology such as an enlarged uterus or myoma
- Failed umbilical or Palmer Approach
- Gynecologic Malignancy

Contraindications: Prior supra-umbilical surgery

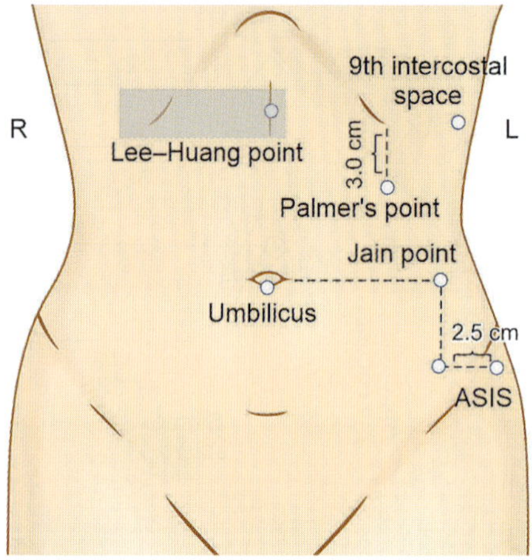

Fig. 8: Lee–Huang point.

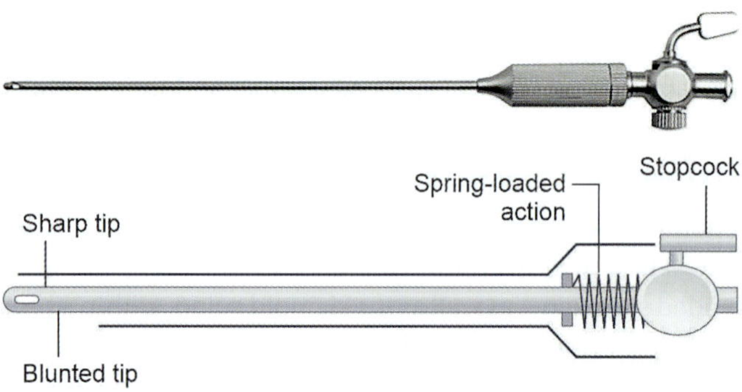

Fig. 9: Veress needle.

CHOOSING THE RIGHT ENTRY METHOD

The choice of access technique must be individualized. No single laparoscopic entry technique has been definitively shown to be safer or superior to the others. Surgeon familiarity, case selection, and patient-specific factors such as body mass index, prior surgeries, and abdominal pathology determine the best approach.

CLOSED ACCESS TECHNIQUE

In closed access technique, pneumoperitoneum is created by Veress needle **(Fig. 9)**.

Before using the Veress needle, its patency and spring mechanism should be verified. Spring action of Veress needle can be checked by pulling the head out.

Steps

See **Figures 10A to D**.

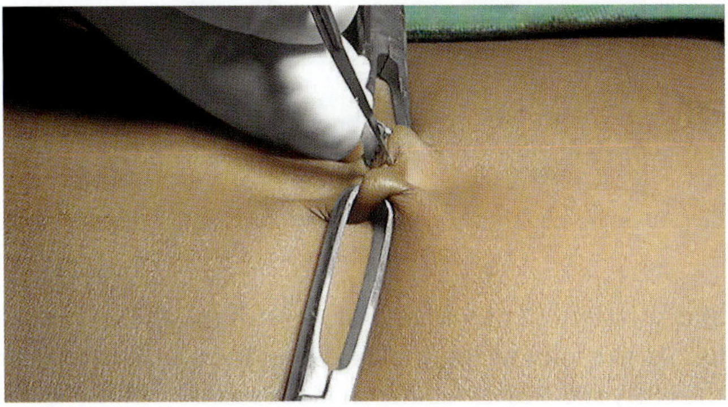

Fig. 10A: 2 mm stab wound over inferior crease of umbilicus.

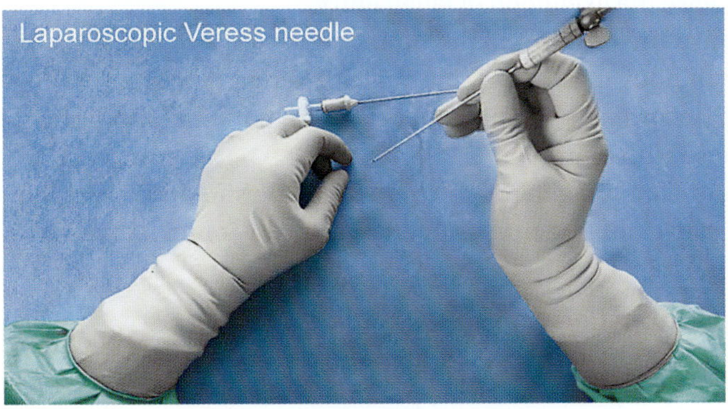

Fig. 10B: Veress needle should be held like a dart.

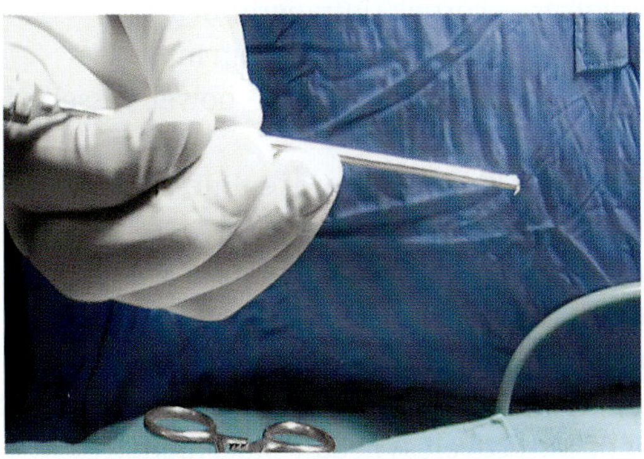

Fig. 10 C: Guard the required length of Veress needle.

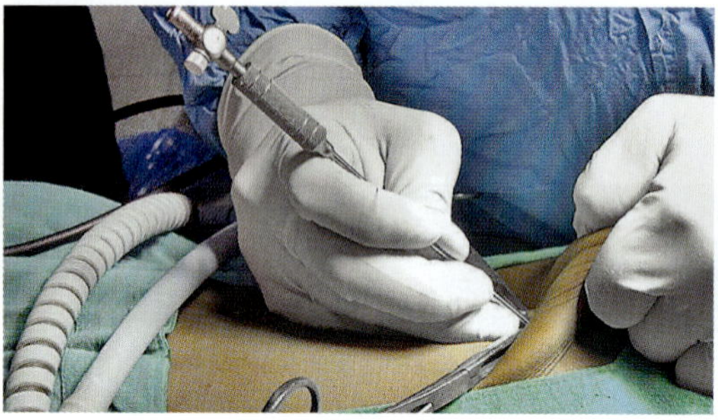

Fig. 10D: Veress Needle should be pointed towards anus but perpendicular to abdominal wall.

Caudal displacement of the umbilicus prior to Veress needle insertion (as described in the Vilos technique) provides an average 6 cm safety margin between the entry site and the common iliac vessels.

Notably, elevating the anterior abdominal wall during Veress needle placement does not reduce the risk of vascular or visceral injury and may, in fact, increase the likelihood of failed entry.

Because the position of the umbilicus relative to the aortic bifurcation varies with body mass index, the angle of Veress needle insertion should be adjusted accordingly—approximately 45° in patients with normal BMI and 90° in those with obesity.

Side-to-side waggling of the Veress needle should be avoided, as it can convert a 1.6 mm puncture into a larger injury of up to 1 cm in viscera or blood vessels.

Tests to Confirm Correct Veress Needle Placement:

- *Irrigation Test:* Inject 5 mL saline with a 10 mL syringe.
  - *Free flow* → needle inside peritoneal cavity.
  - *Resistance* → incorrect placement.
- *Aspiration Test:* Try to aspirate the injected saline.
  - *No fluid returns* → correct (intraperitoneal).
  - *Fluid returns* → preperitoneal or organ injury.
  - *Fecal matter, blood, or excess fluid* → bowel, vessel, or bladder injury/ascites.
- *Hanging Drop Test:* Place a drop of saline on the needle hub; lift the abdominal wall **(Fig. 11A)**.
  - *Drop sucked in* → correct placement (negative intraabdominal pressure).
- *Intraperitoneal Pressure Test:*
  - An intraperitoneal pressure of less than 10 mm Hg is a reliable indicator of correct Veress needle placement.

Saline Test: Withdraw, Instill, Withdraw (Fig. 11B)

Saline test not 100% accurate

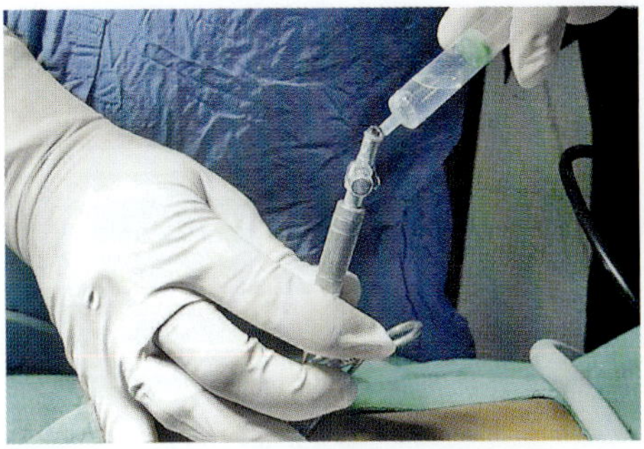

Fig. 11A: Hanging drop test.

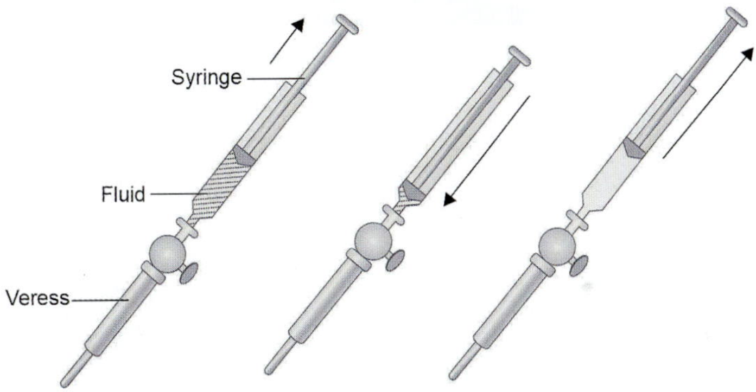

Fig. 11B: Saline test.

CONFIRMING PROPER PLACEMENT AND INSUFFLATION (FIG. 12)

After confirming correct intraperitoneal placement, carbon dioxide insufflation should be initiated gradually.

- Set the pressure cutoff to 20–25 mm Hg
- Begin insufflation at a low flow rate (≈1 L/min)
- Ensure gas entry occurs at a low pressure (<8 mm Hg)
- After 0.5 L of insufflation, the flow rate can be increased
- Continue insufflation until the pressure reaches the set cutoff (20–25 mm Hg)
- Symmetrical distension of the abdomen and tympanic note on percussion confirm adequate pneumoperitoneum
- An intra-abdominal pressure of 20–25 mm Hg should be achieved before inserting the primary trocar **(Fig. 13)**.
- The primary trocar is then introduced in a controlled manner, ideally under direct vision. Once the laparoscope is inserted, the peritoneal cavity should be inspected immediately for any evidence of bleeding, bowel injury, or unusual adhesions.
- Trocar and cannula should be held like a piston **(Fig. 14A)**

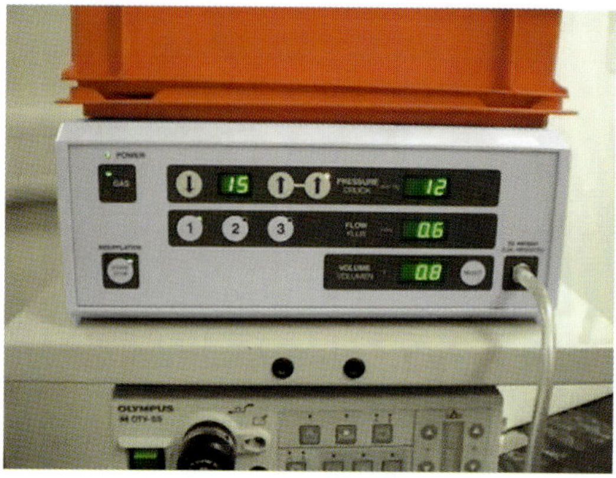

Fig. 12: Insufflator device.

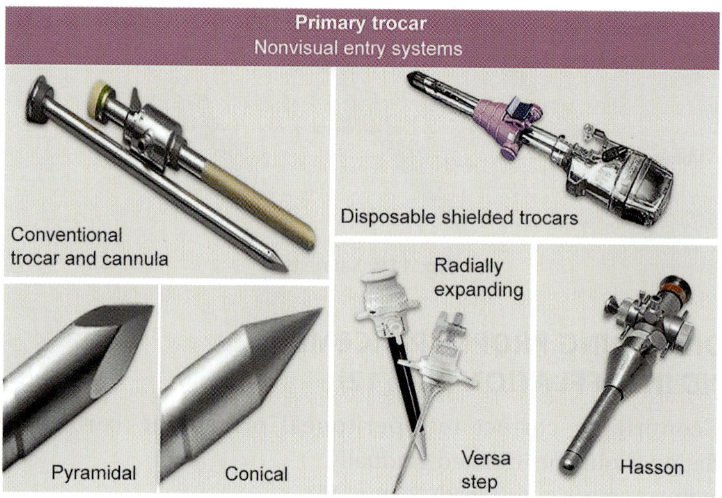

Fig. 13: Types of primary trocars.

- Trocar insertion by a screwing motion **(Fig. 14B)**
- The primary trocar should be inserted at 90° to the skin, through the incision at the base of the umbilicus
- Once the laparoscope has been introduced it should be rotated through 360° to check for any adherent bowel
- The risk of bowel injury decreases with larger gas insufflation and greater abdominal wall tension **(Figs. 16A and B)**.

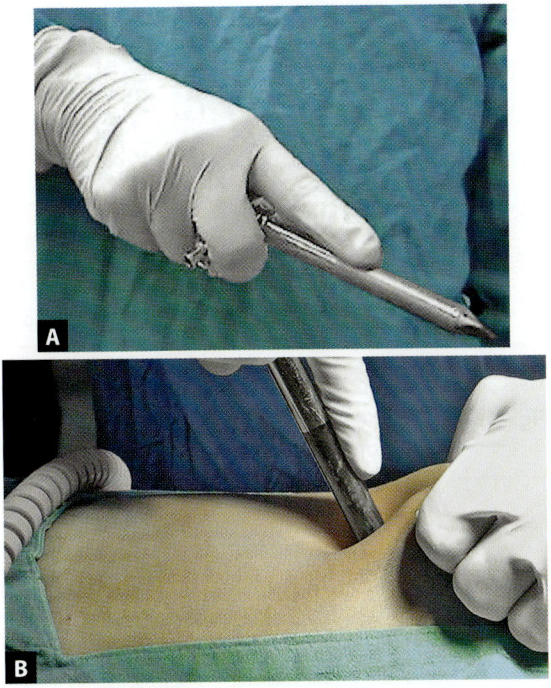

Figs. 14A and B: (A) Trocar and cannula should be held like a piston; and (B) Trocar insertion by a screwing motion.

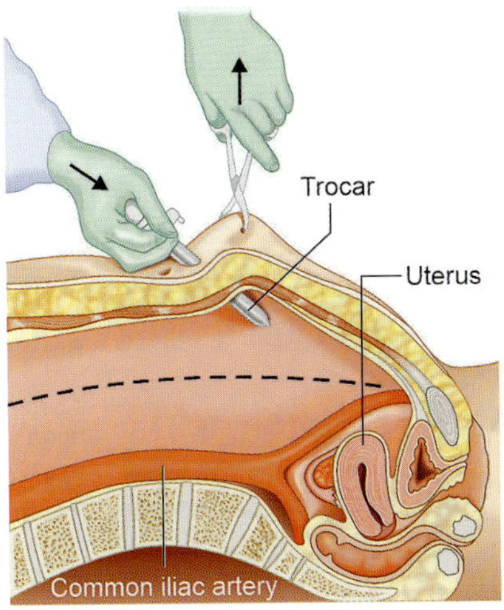

Fig. 15: Trocar insertion.

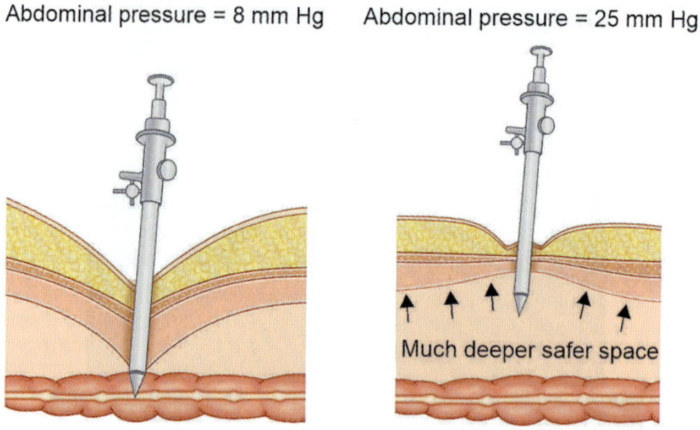

Figs. 16A and B: (A) Abdominal pressure = 8 mm Hg; and (B) Abdominal pressure = 25 mm Hg.

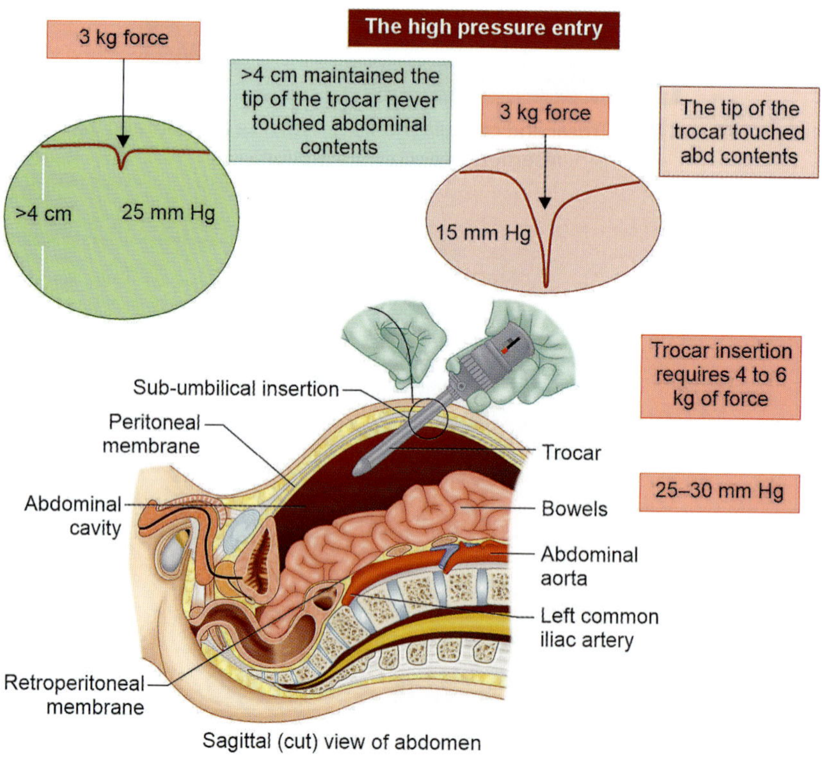

Fig. 17: *Contd…*

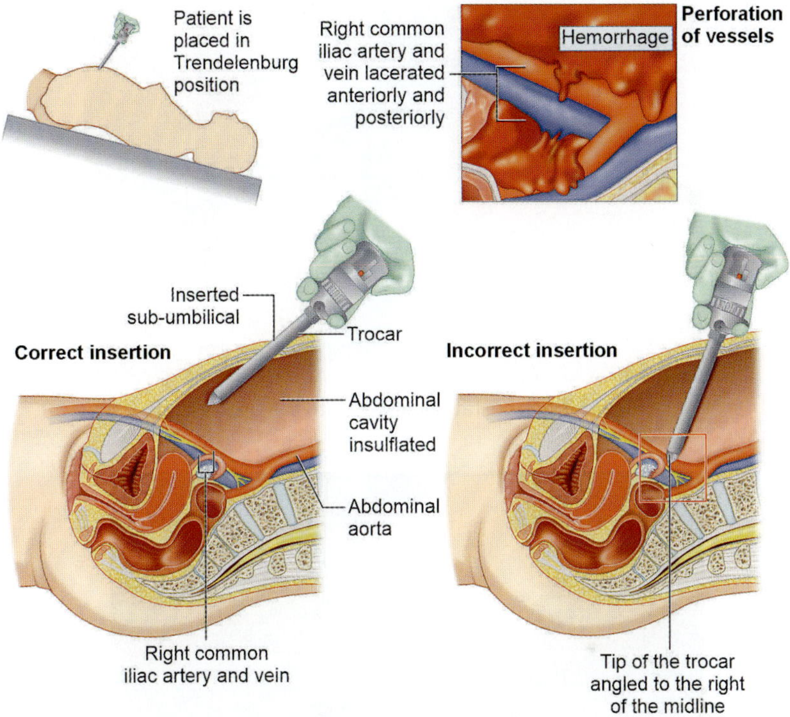

Fig. 17: Force during Trocar insertion.

OPEN (HASSON) TECHNIQUE

See **Figures 18A to F**.

Steps

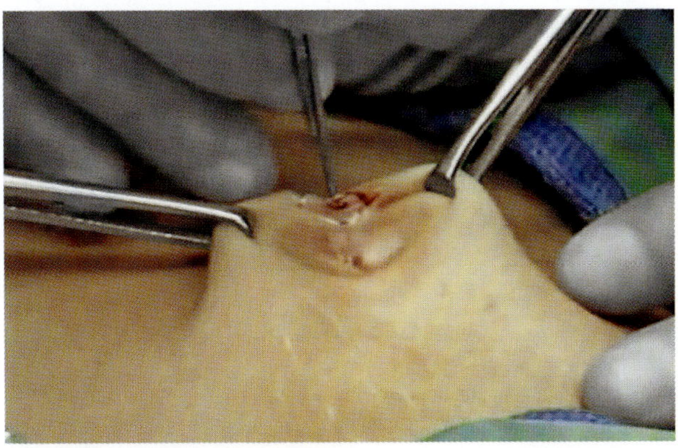

Fig. 18A: Skin Incision for open technique.

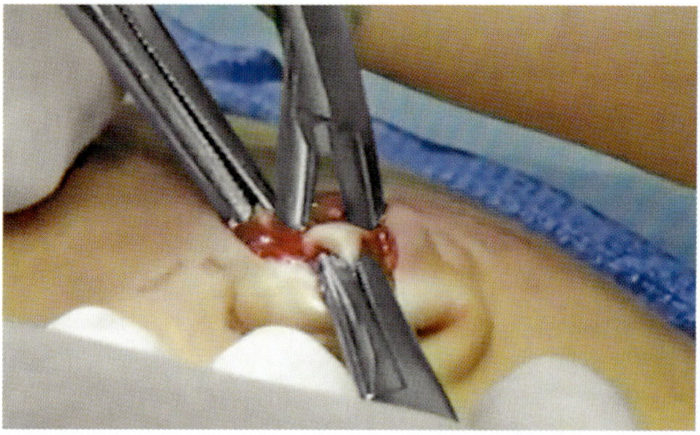

Fig. 18B: Hemostat is stabbed into the peritoneum.

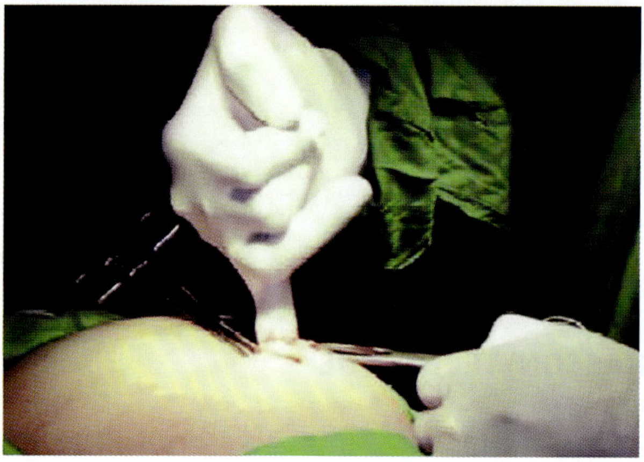

Fig. 18C: Digital exploration following open access can help identify adhesions (Outer view).

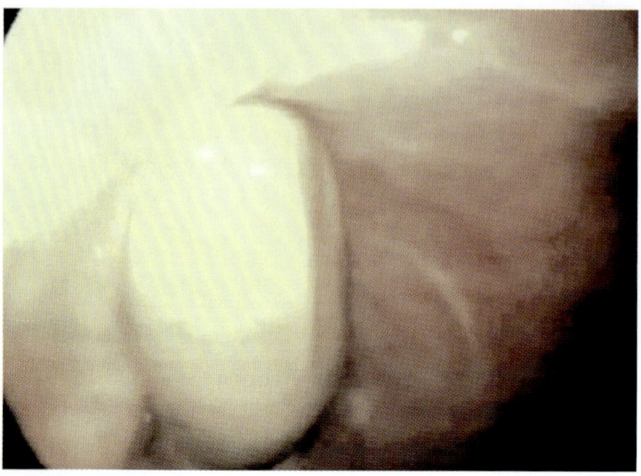

Fig. 18D: Digital exploration following open access can help identify adhesions (Inner view).

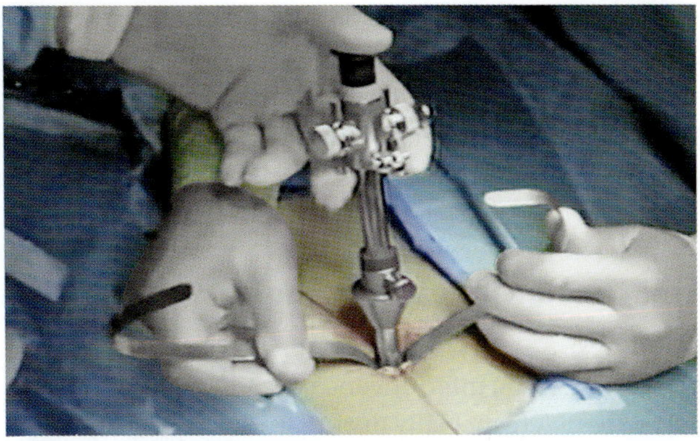

Fig. 18E: Insertion of the Hasson trocar.

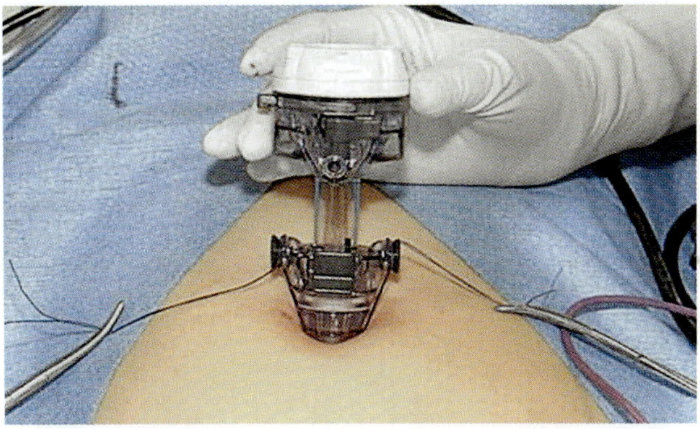

Fig. 18F: Securing the Hasson Trocar.

- Skin Incision for Open Technique
- The hemostat is stabbed into the peritoneum
- Digital exploration following open access can help identify adhesions.
- Insertion of the Hasson trocar
- Securing the Hasson Trocar

SECONDARY PORTS

Secondary ports are inserted under direct vision, and any inadvertent injury caused during their placement may be considered negligent.

Principles

- Avoid injury to the inferior epigastric vessels
- Prevent bowel and vascular injury
- Minimize the risk of port-site hernia

Technique

Secondary ports should be inserted under direct vision, perpendicular to the skin, with a pneumoperitoneum pressure of 20–25 mm Hg. Once the trocar penetrates the peritoneum, it should be angled toward the anterior pelvis.

Proper placement of the secondary trocars under laparoscopic guidance is essential to avoid injury to inferior epigastric vessels. Continuous vigilance during this phase significantly reduces the risk of complications **(Figs. 19A and B)**.

Injuries Associated with Laparoscopic Entry

- *Vascular Injuries:*
    - *Major vessels:* Aorta, inferior vena cava, iliac vessels.
    - *Epigastric vessels* (especially during trocar insertion).
- Visceral Injuries:
    - *Bowel injury:* Small or large intestine.
    - *Bladder injury:* Particularly in patients with previous pelvic surgery.
    - *Stomach or omental injury* (rare).
- *Abdominal Wall Injuries:*
    - *Bleeding or hematoma* from inferior epigastric vessels.
    - *Nerve injury:* Ilioinguinal, iliohypogastric, or genitofemoral nerves.

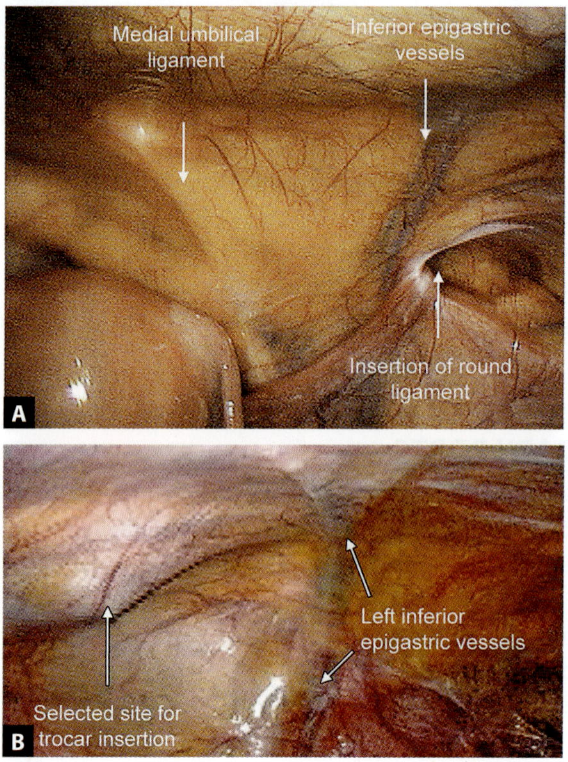

Figs. 19A and B: Secondary port placement site relation with major abdominal structures.

KEY POINTS

- Safe abdominal entry remains the cornerstone of laparoscopic safety. Most access-related complications are preventable with proper patient selection, meticulous technique, and adherence to anatomical principles. The surgeon should be proficient with more than one entry method and capable of modifying the approach depending on individual patient factors.
- The umbilicus remains the standard entry site, but Palmer's and Jain's points offer reliable alternatives in patients with previous surgery or altered anatomy. Adequate decompression of viscera, correct insertion angle, and verification of pneumoperitoneum are non-negotiable steps for every laparoscopic case.
- A clear backup plan, availability of appropriate equipment, and immediate recognition of complications define surgical preparedness. Above all, patience, precision, and respect for the anatomy ensure that the benefits of laparoscopy are achieved without compromising safety.

SUGGESTED READING

1. Anandhi V, Rajeswari K, Jebakani CF. A study of the origin and course of the inferior epigastric artery and its significance in laparoscopic surgery. IJAR. 2016;4(3.2):2692-7.
2. Djokovic D, Gupta J, Thomas V, Maher P, Ternamian A, Vilos G, et al. Principles of safe laparoscopic entry. Eur J Obstet Gynecol Reprod Biol. 2016;201:179-88.
3. Jain N, Jain V, Agarwal C, Bansal P, Gupta S, Bansal B. Left Lateral Port: Safe Laparoscopic Port Entry in Previous Large Upper Abdomen Laparotomy Scar. J Minim Invasive Gynecol. 2019;26(5):973-6.
4. Jain N, Srivastava S, Bayya SLP, Jain V. Jain point laparoscopic entry in contraindications of Palmers point. Front Surg. 2022;9:928081.
5. Raimondo D, Raffone A, Travaglino A, Ferla S, Maletta M, Rovero G, et al. Laparoscopic entry techniques: Which should you prefer? Int J Gynecology Obstet. 2023;160(3):742-50.
6. Recknagel JD, Goodman LR. Clinical Perspective Concerning Abdominal Entry Techniques. J Minim Invasive Gynecol. 2021;28(3):467-74.
7. Thepsuwan J, Huang KG, Wilamarta M, Adlan AS, Manvelyan V, Lee CL. Principles of safe abdominal entry in laparoscopic gynecologic surgery. Gynecol Minim Invasive Ther. 2013;2(4):105-9.
8. Vilos G, Vilos A, Jacob GP, Abu-Rafea B, Ternamian A. Safe Veress Needle Intraperitoneal Placement and Safer Laparoscopic Entry. J Minim Invasive Gynecol. 2018;25(7):1137.
9. Vilos GA, Ternamian A, Laberge PY, Vilos AG, Abu-Rafea B, Scattolon S, et al. Guideline No. 412: Laparoscopic Entry for Gynaecological Surgery. J Obstet Gynaecol Can. 2021;43(3):376-389.e1.

10 CHAPTER

Laparoscopic Evaluation of Fertility

Abhinibesh Chatterjee

INTRODUCTION

Infertility is defined as the inability to conceive after 12 months of regular, unprotected intercourse. It affects 10–15% of couples globally. Pelvic factors such as tubal block, endometriosis, pelvic inflammatory disease (PID), genital tuberculosis (GTB), adhesions and pelvic anatomical abnormalities contribute to nearly 35–40% of female infertility. Laparoscopy provides a direct, panoramic view of the pelvic organs and allows simultaneous diagnosis and treatment of intra-abdominal causes of infertility. It is therefore regarded as the gold standard in the evaluation of tubal and peritoneal factors.

WHY LAPAROSCOPY IN INFERTILITY?

Direct visualization of uterus, ovaries, fallopian tubes and peritoneum

- Detects lesions not seen on ultrasound or hysterosalpingography (HSG)
- Enables chromopertubation—the most reliable test for tubal patency
- Diagnostic + therapeutic in the same sitting (endometriosis, adhesiolysis, cystectomy, etc.)
- Improves natural conception rates and helps in planning IVF/ICSI

INDICATIONS FOR DIAGNOSTIC LAPAROSCOPY IN INFERTILITY

Primary or secondary infertility ≥1 year

- Abnormal HSG: Hydrosalpinx, tubal block
- Unexplained infertility after normal semen analysis and ovulation status
- Suspected endometriosis/chronic pelvic pain/dyspareunia
- History of PID, tuberculosis, ectopic pregnancy, pelvic surgery
- Evaluation before IVF in selected patients (hydrosalpinx, severe endometriosis)

PREOPERATIVE EVALUATION

History: Menstrual pattern, dysmenorrhea, dyspareunia, past surgeries, PID, TB

Clinical examination: Uterine mobility, adnexal masses, tenderness

Investigations:

Semen analysis of male partner

- *Hormonal profile:* AMH, FSH, LH, TSH, prolactin
- *Ultrasound pelvis:* Uterus, endometrium, ovarian reserve
- HSG for tubal lumen but limited in peritoneal pathology

Consent: Must include possibility of operative procedures and complications.

SURGICAL SETUP AND INSTRUMENTATION

General anesthesia

- Lithotomy position with Trendelenburg tilt
- Foley catheterization
- Creation of pneumoperitoneum using Veress needle or open (Hasson) method
- Ports: 10 mm umbilical port (camera)
- 5 mm ports in left and right iliac fossae

Instruments: Telescope (30°), atraumatic graspers, scissors, suction-irrigation, bipolar/monopolar cautery.

STEPWISE PROCEDURE OF LAPAROSCOPIC EVALUATION (TABLE 1)

1. Entry and survey of abdomen
2. Inspection of uterus: Size, shape, fibroids, anomalies
3. Inspection of ovaries: Size, follicular pattern, cysts, PCOS, endometriomas
4. Fallopian tubes: Course, fimbrial ends, mobility
5. Pouch of Douglas, uterosacral ligaments, ovarian fossa
6. Chromopertubation: Methylene blue dye is injected via an intrauterine cannula; dye spill through fimbrial ends indicates tubal patency
7. Documentation of any pathology through images/video

Normal Laparoscopic Findings

See **Table 1**.

TABLE 1: Normal laparoscopic findings.

Structure	*Normal findings*
Uterus	Normal size, smooth surface, mobile
Ovaries	Normal volume with follicles; no cysts or adhesions
Fallopian Tubes	Free, pink, delicate fimbriae; bilateral dye spill
Peritoneum	Shiny, avascular, no implants
Pouch of Douglas	Deep, free of adhesions

Abnormal Findings and Pathologies

1. Endometriosis **(Fig. 1)**
   - Chronic estrogen-dependent inflammatory condition with endometrial-like tissue outside uterus
   - *Common sites:* Ovaries, uterosacral ligaments, pouch of Douglas
   - *Laparoscopic findings:* Powder-burn lesions, red/yellow implants, endometriomas, adhesions
   - *Treatment:* Ablation/excision of lesions, adhesiolysis, endometriotic cystectomy
2. Pelvic Adhesions **(Fig. 2)**
   - Result from PID, tuberculosis, endometriosis, previous surgery
   - Appear as filmy or dense fibrous bands fixing tubes or ovaries
   - Lead to restricted tubal motility and impaired ovum pickup
   - *Treatment:* Laparoscopic adhesiolysis with sharp/blunt dissection or energy devices

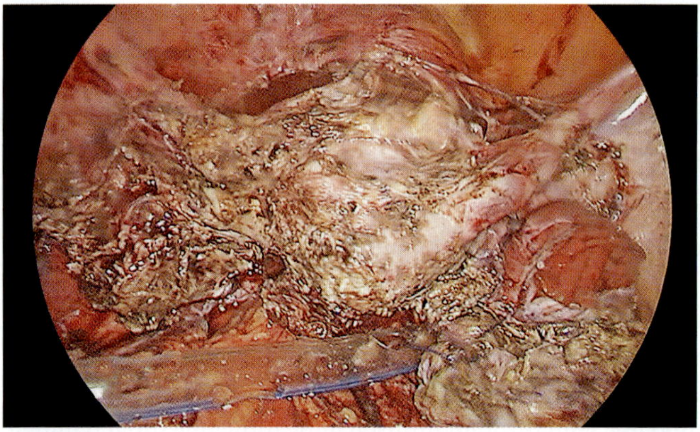

Fig. 1: Endometriosis.

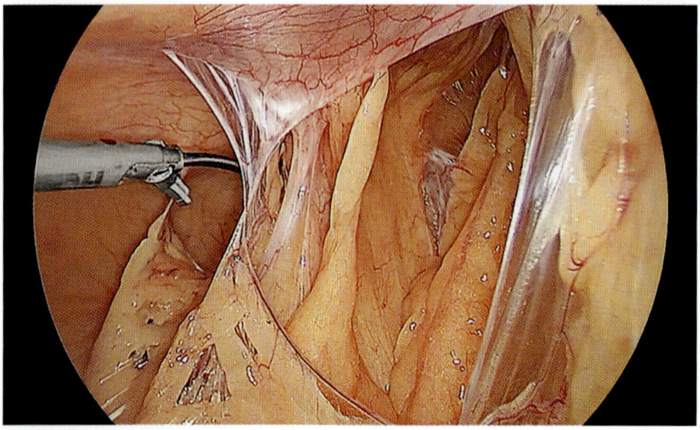

Fig. 2: Pelvic adhesions in endometriosis.

3. Tubal Block/Hydrosalpinx
   - Proximal or distal block may be visualized during chromopertubation **(Fig. 3)**
   - *Hydrosalpinx:* Dilated fluid-filled tube with clubbed fimbriae
   - *Management:* Tubal cannulation **(Fig. 4)**, Fimbrioplasty, salpingostomy, or salpingectomy pre-IVF (to improve implantation)
4. Polycystic Ovary Syndrome (PCOS)
   - Enlarged ovaries with multiple peripheral follicles (>12, "string of pearls")
   - Thickened capsule, increased stroma
   - In clomiphene-resistant cases, laparoscopic ovarian drilling is an option **(Fig. 5)**

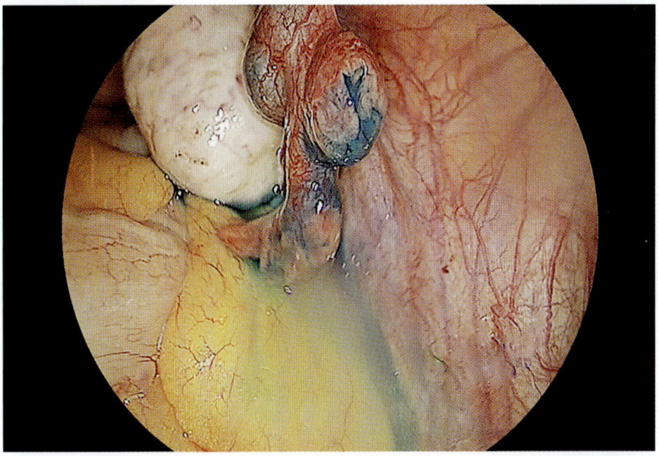

Fig. 3: Chromopertubation.

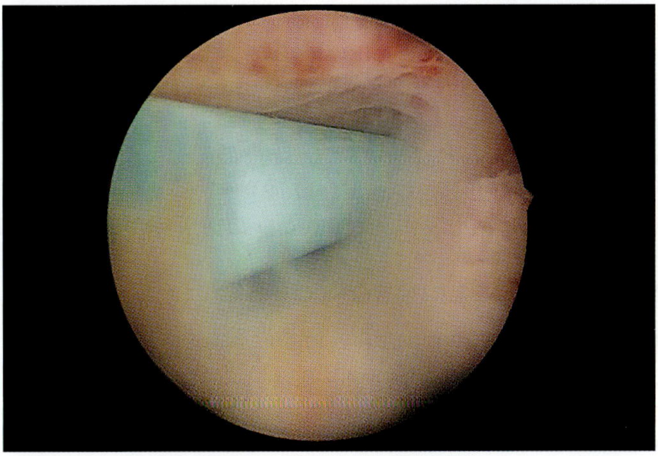

Fig. 4: Tubal cannulation.

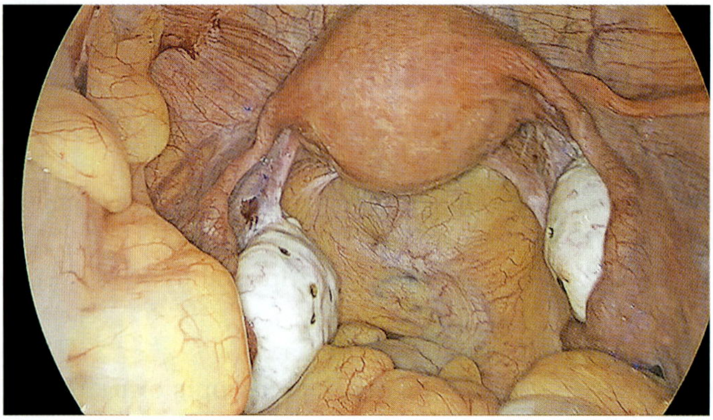

Fig. 5: Laparoscopic ovarian drilling.

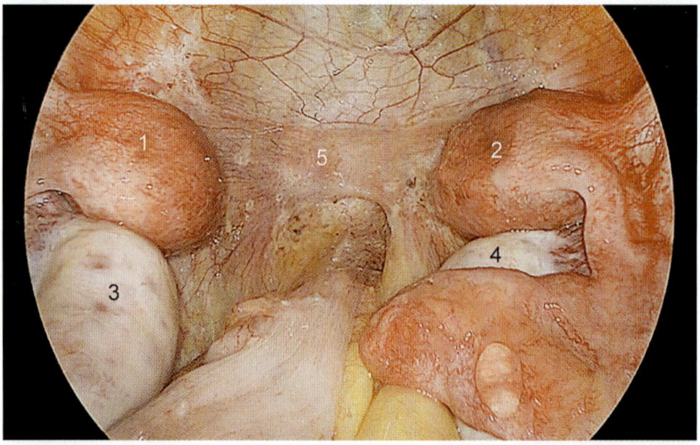

Fig. 6: MRKH syndrome showing (1) left uterine horn, (2) right uterine horn, (3) left ovary, (4) right ovary, and (5) peritoneal plate.

5. Genital Tuberculosis
   - Seen in high-prevalence countries like India
   - *Findings:* Streaked tubes, beaded appearance, tubercles on peritoneum, caseous nodules
   - Adhesions are dense, tubo-ovarian masses may be present
6. Müllerian Anomalies **(Fig. 6 and Table 2)**

*Laparoscopy + hysteroscopy are used together to differentiate **(Table 2)***

ADVANTAGES OF LAPAROSCOPY

- Gold standard for evaluating tubal patency and pelvic pathology
- Diagnostic + therapeutic in one sitting
- Short hospital stay and faster recovery
- Helps decide need for IUI vs IVF
- Avoids unnecessary IVF in correctable condition

TABLE 2: Laparoscopic findings in Mullerian anomalies.

Anomaly	*Laparoscopic findings*
Septate uterus	Normal external fundus
Bicornuate uterus	Two separate horns with fundal cleft
Unicornuate uterus	One rudimentary horn or absent one side

LIMITATIONS AND RISKS

Invasive procedure under anesthesia

- *Complications:* Bowel, bladder or vascular injury (<1%)
- Tubal spasm may cause false tubal block
- Requires surgical expertise and equipment
- Not first-line in young patients with <3 years infertility and no risk factors

KEY POINTS

Laparoscopy plays a pivotal role in the evaluation of female infertility, especially when pelvic, tubal or peritoneal factors are suspected. It enables direct visualization of the uterus, tubes, ovaries and peritoneum and is the most accurate method for assessing tubal patency through chromopertubation. Common conditions diagnosed include endometriosis, adhesions, hydrosalpinx, PCOS and genital tuberculosis. Its greatest advantage is the ability to diagnose and treat in the same sitting. However, laparoscopy must be performed after basic infertility evaluation and should be reserved for appropriate indications rather than as a routine first-line test. In experienced hands, it improves fertility outcomes, guides ART decisions and prevents unnecessary IVF. Proper patient selection, counseling and surgical precision are essential for best results.

SUGGESTED READING

1. ASRM Practice Committee. Fertil Steril. 2021;116(6):e1-e16.
2. Camus M, Poncelet C, Goffinet F, Wainer B, Merlet F, Nisand I, et al. Pregnancy rates after in-vitro fertilization in cases of tubal infertility with and without hydrosalpinx: a meta-analysis of published comparative studies. Hum Reprod. 1999;14(6):1243-9.
3. Chapron C, Querleu D, Bruhat MA, Madelenat P, Fernandez H, Pierre F, et al. Surgical complications of diagnostic and operative gynaecological laparoscopy: a series of 29,966 cases. Hum Reprod. 1998;13(4):867-72.
4. Fauque P, et al. Hum Reprod. 2020;35(4):876-84.
5. Johnson N, et al. Cochrane Database Syst Rev. 2019;(3):CD001398.
6. Practice Committee of ESHRE. Hum Reprod. 2022;37(5):855-81.
7. Sharma JB. Int J Gynaecol Obstet. 2015;129(2):146-51.

11 CHAPTER

Laparoscopic Tissue Retrieval Techniques

Dinesh Kansal, Supriya Mahipal, Yamini Kansal

INTRODUCTION

Minimally invasive surgery has transformed gynecologic practice by enabling reduced postoperative pain, faster recovery, minimal scarring, and enhanced cosmetic outcomes. However, these advantages can be compromised when surgical incisions need to be extended for specimen removal. As a result, specimen retrieval has emerged as a critical technical and oncologic challenge in both laparoscopic and robotic procedures. An ideal retrieval strategy must allow complete and safe extraction of the specimen while preventing intraoperative spillage and preserving tissue integrity for accurate histopathological assessment, especially when malignancy is suspected **(Fig. 1)**. Over the years, a range of minimally invasive retrieval routes and technologies—including containment systems, specialized retrieval bags, and natural orifice extraction techniques—have been developed to address these complexities. The choice of technique depends on multiple factors, including specimen size, consistency, suspected pathology, and the need to uphold strict oncologic safety.

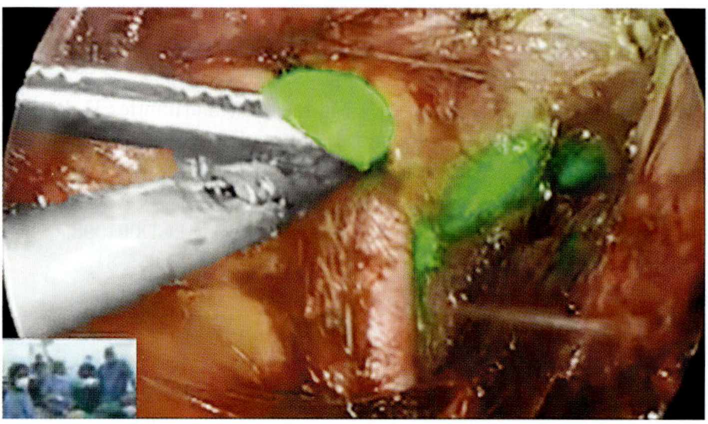

Fig. 1: Sentinel node in endometrial cancer.

TECHNIQUES FOR LAPAROSCOPIC TISSUE RETRIEVAL

Direct Extraction through the 10 mm Cannula

Small specimens such as tissue from prophylactic salpingectomy, small fibroids, adenomyomectomy fragments **(Figs. 2 and 3)**, tubal ectopic pregnancy **(Fig. 4)**, para-ovarian or fimbrial cysts, peritoneal biopsies, and sentinel lymph nodes in endometrial carcinoma can be removed directly through a 10–12 mm port using grasper forceps. Slightly larger benign specimens, such as an endometriotic cyst wall, may be elongated using a Z-technique **(Fig. 3)** with scissors or an energy device under direct vision to facilitate removal without enlarging the incision. Importantly, no specimen should be extracted directly through the skin incision without protection, as this may increase the risk of port-site implantation of cells, leading to complications such as scar endometriosis, myomatosis, or mucinous

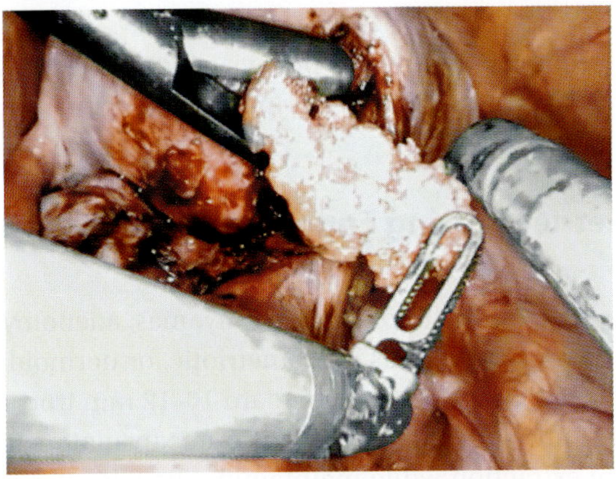

Fig. 2: Strips of adenomyotic tissue in robotic surgery

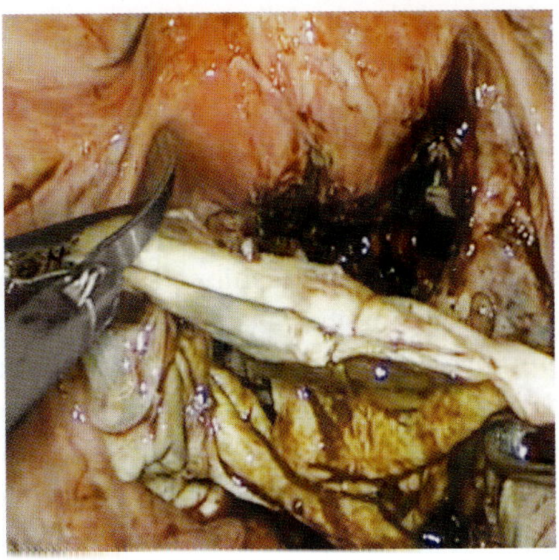

Fig. 3: Endometriotic cyst elongated by Z technique

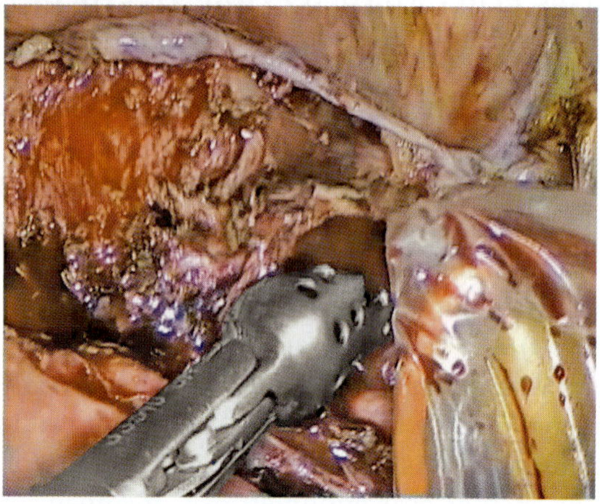

Fig. 4: Friable RPOC from scar ectopic being kept in endobag

cystadenoma seeding. Continuous port visualization during extraction is essential to prevent port-site injury, tearing of the specimen, and inadvertent tissue loss.

Specimen Retrieval Using Endoscopic Retrieval Bags (Endobags)

Large specimens such as multiple or giant myomas, adenomyotic uteri, and adnexal cysts (serous, mucinous, endometriotic, or dermoid) are often too large to be removed intact through standard 10–12 mm trocars. Endoscopic retrieval bags (Endobags) are designed to encapsulate such specimens, allowing secure extraction while maintaining the advantages of minimally invasive surgery. Their use has been shown to reduce contamination, port-site recurrence, and intra-abdominal dissemination of cyst contents.

Endobags may be commercially manufactured or indigenously prepared. Commercial retrieval systems are typically made of impermeable, tear-resistant materials and incorporate closing mechanisms such as zip-locks or metal wire drawstrings, allowing secure sealing before exteriorization. However, very large specimens may not fit within standard commercial bags. In such situations, indigenous bags fashioned by the surgeon using sterile surgical gloves or polythene pouches available in the operating theatre (e.g., urobags) can be employed. When using these improvised bags, additional caution is required due to their greater risk of rupture. A purse-string suture is often placed at the open end before introducing the bag to reinforce closure. These self-made retrieval systems are commonly utilized for adnexal masses including dermoid cysts **(Fig. 5)** and solid ovarian tumors.

The Endo bag is typically introduced through a 10 mm lower abdominal port, opened intra-abdominally, and the specimen placed within it. The

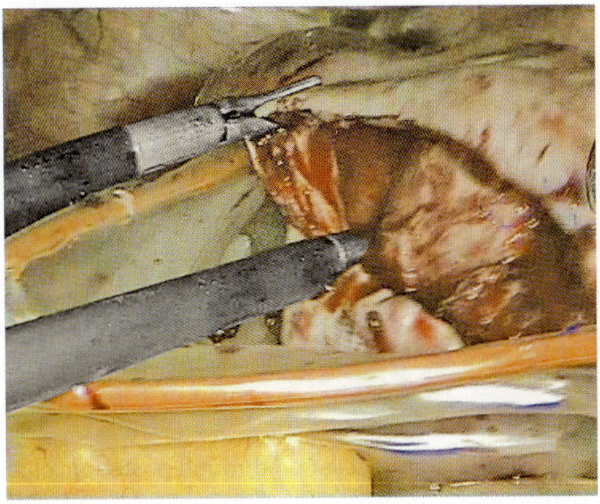

Fig. 5: Dermoid cystectomy being done within endobag

mouth of the bag is then exteriorized and held wide open. The bag is gently pulled towards the abdominal wall, and a controlled nick is made over the cyst using a stab knife to facilitate decompression. After suctioning the cyst contents, removal is aided by traction with forceps. All steps must be performed under laparoscopic visualization to minimize the risk of bag rupture, intraperitoneal spillage, and inadvertent injury to internal organs. During dermoid cystectomy, in-bag cystectomy may be performed from the outset to prevent spillage. The ovary containing the cyst is placed within the bag, and cystectomy is completed entirely inside it.

The end bag should be inspected for integrity both before and after extraction, and the retrieval site should be securely closed, often using a cobbler's needle technique, to prevent postoperative port-site hernia. When only 5 mm ancillary ports are used, the umbilical port may serve as the retrieval site using a railroading technique.

Transvaginal Extraction

Transvaginal natural orifice specimen extraction (v-NOSE) combines laparoscopic surgery with vaginal retrieval to permit scarless specimen removal, resulting in reduced postoperative pain and improved cosmetic outcomes. In total laparoscopic hysterectomy (TLH), specimens are routinely extracted transvaginally, and if required, coring, bisection, or piecemeal morcellation may be performed to facilitate removal. Specimens from laparoscopic radical hysterectomy, including lymph nodes and omentum, can be collected in an Endo bag and removed intact through the vagina, maintaining oncological safety.

A posterior colpotomy provides a natural access route for specimen retrieval during uterus-preserving procedures such as myomectomy, ovarian cystectomy, or oophorectomy. The colpotomy incision is made on the

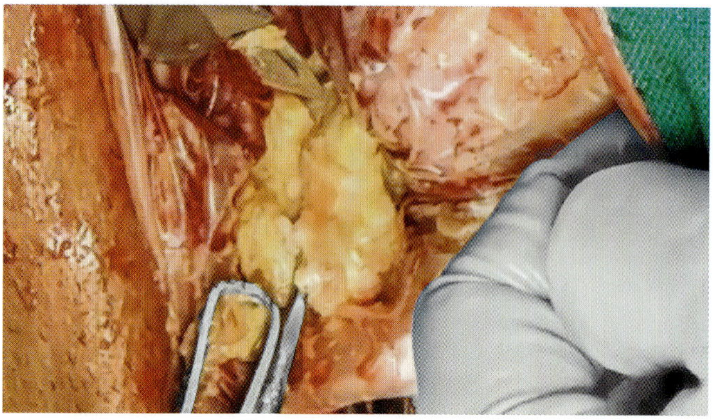

Fig. 6: Vaginal in-bag morcellation through posterior colpotomy

posterior vaginal wall between the uterosacral ligaments, guided by a vaginal tube or sponge holder to maintain pneumoperitoneum and ensure proper localization. In patients with rectovaginal adhesions, careful rectal dissection may be necessary prior to creating the colpotomy to avoid rectal injury **(Fig. 6)**.

During extraction, the vaginal assistant holds the mouth of the Endo bag containing the specimen or myoma under direct laparoscopic visualization using a grasper. Following specimen removal, the colpotomy incision is closed laparoscopically with 1-0 Vicryl. This approach eliminates the need to enlarge an abdominal port site for larger specimens and offers the added advantage of allowing intact specimen removal without fragmentation, thereby reducing the risk of spillage, and preserving tissue integrity for histopathological evaluation.

Contained Tissue Morcellation (In-Bag Morcellation)

Contained, or "in-bag," morcellation has become the preferred method for extracting large specimens in minimally invasive gynecologic surgery. In this technique, the excised tissue is placed within a sealed containment bag introduced laparoscopically, and morcellation is performed entirely inside the bag. Multiple studies have demonstrated that contained morcellation significantly reduces distant tissue dissemination and intra-abdominal contamination, thereby enhancing oncologic safety.

Manual Morcellation

Manual morcellation involves fragmenting the specimen within a containment system using scissors or an energy device such as a harmonic scalpel. This technique is cost-effective and widely accessible, particularly in resource-limited settings. However, it may be time-consuming for very large or firm specimens and requires meticulous laparoscopic monitoring to avoid bag damage and spillage.

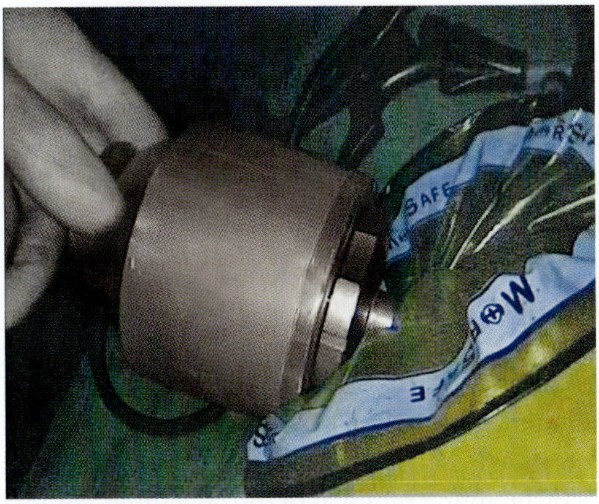

Fig. 7: Power morcellator introduced through the Morsafe bag

Power Morcellation

Power morcellation merits special consideration. Solid specimens such as myomas or subtotal hysterectomy specimens often require morcellation into long strips for removal through small ports. Electronic power morcellators allow rapid fragmentation and extraction of large tissue volumes while maintaining minimally invasive access. These devices consist of a motor-driven rotating cutting tube controlled by foot or hand activation, with a blunt obturator to prevent injury during insertion. Commercially available containment bags for power morcellation are offered in various sizes. After the specimen is placed within the bag, the telescope and morcellator are introduced into the bag, and a secondary insufflated cavity is created to provide working space. The morcellator is usually introduced through the left lower port. Adjustable speed and rotational direction enable precise control by the surgeon, while continuous visualization of the morcellator blade during gradual traction minimizes the risk of injury and surgical complications.

The motorized cutting action facilitates efficient removal of large tissue masses while preserving tissue architecture for histopathological evaluation. It is now considered mandatory to perform power morcellation within a containment system such as Morsafe **(Fig. 7)**, to prevent high-velocity tissue dissemination in cases of unsuspected leiomyosarcoma or subsequent development of multiple peritoneal myomatosis.

LAPAROSCOPICALLY-ASSISTED MYOMECTOMY

In laparoscopically assisted myomectomy (LAM), the fibroid is enucleated laparoscopically and then removed through a small low transverse abdominal incision. The uterus can be exteriorized through this incision, allowing convenient suturing of the myomectomy sites. This approach reduces operating time and enhances safety, particularly when the surgeon has limited experience in advanced laparoscopic suturing techniques.

MINI LAPAROTOMY OR PORT-SITE EXTENSION

For large or potentially malignant specimens, a small suprapubic transverse mini-laparotomy, or controlled enlargement of an existing port site, allows intact specimen removal while still preserving many of the advantages of minimally invasive surgery. This approach is particularly valuable in cases involving a markedly enlarged uterus in endometrial carcinoma or ovarian masses with uncertain pathology, where contained extraction may be technically challenging or ontologically inadvisable.

Mini-laparotomy provides a balance between minimal access and oncologic safety by enabling removal of the specimen without morcellation, thereby avoiding tissue fragmentation, spillage, or compromise of histopathological assessment. The incision can often be limited to 3–5 cm and placed cosmetically in the suprapubic region, maintaining favorable postoperative recovery, reduced pain, and shorter hospital stay compared with traditional laparotomy.

ONCOLOGIC CONSIDERATIONS

In cases of suspected or confirmed malignancy, strict adherence to oncologic principles is essential during specimen retrieval to prevent tumor dissemination and ensure accurate staging. Intact specimen retrieval is critical for precise staging in ovarian, endometrial, and cervical cancers, as fragmentation may compromise pathological evaluation and influence treatment planning. Hence, vaginal extraction or mini-laparotomy are preferred methods for intact removal. Although uncommon, port-site metastasis remains a recognized complication of minimally invasive oncologic surgery, with increased risk when tissue spillage or peritoneal contamination occurs. Inspecting and irrigating port sites after specimen retrieval to minimize the risk of tumor cell seeding is mandatory. Careful technique, appropriate use of containment systems, and vigilant port-site management are therefore fundamental to maintaining oncologic safety.

CONCLUSION

Specimen retrieval remains one of the most demanding steps in laparoscopic and robotic surgery, requiring a balance between technical feasibility and oncologic prudence. Innovations such as advanced containment systems, improved retrieval bags, and transvaginal or natural-orifice extraction have expanded the possibilities for safe and effective removal of even large or complex specimens without sacrificing the benefits of a minimally invasive approach. Individualizing the retrieval method—while rigorously adhering to containment principles, avoiding tissue fragmentation in cases of suspected malignancy, and ensuring meticulous port-site management—is essential to minimize spillage and postoperative complications. As technology and surgical expertise continue to advance, specimen retrieval techniques will evolve further toward safer, more efficient, and cosmetically superior outcomes, ensuring that minimally invasive surgery retains its therapeutic advantages while upholding the highest standards of patient safety.

KEY POINTS

- *Tissue retrieval is the final, crucial step* in laparoscopic surgery—where surgical precision meets oncologic responsibility.
- The chosen technique must ensure *complete removal, secure containment, and preservation of specimen integrity.*
- *Endobags, in-bag morcellation, and transvaginal extraction (v-NOSE)* are key advancements enabling safe, scarless, and efficient specimen retrieval.
- Use of *containment systems* prevents spillage, minimizes the risk of chemical peritonitis, and safeguards against port-site metastasis.
- *Direct visualization and meticulous handling* during extraction reduce the likelihood of intra-abdominal injury or tissue loss.
- *Port closure after retrieval is mandatory* to prevent postoperative herniation.
- Technique selection should be individualized based on *specimen size, pathology, and malignancy risk.*
- The guiding principle for every laparoscopic surgeon: *"Remove completely, contain safely, and close securely."*
- Mastery of retrieval techniques defines not just surgical skill—but surgical wisdom and safety.

SUGGESTED READING

1. Kho KA, Nezhat C. Evaluating the risks of electric uterine morcellation. JAMA. 2016;316(9):905-6.
2. Nezhat C, Li A, Abed S, Balassiano E, Soliemannjad R, Nezhat A. Minimally invasive surgery in gynecology: past, present, and future. J Minim Invasive Gynecol. 2019;26(1):5-18
3. Parker WH, Fu YS, Berek JS. Uterine sarcoma in patients undergoing minimally invasive gynecologic surgery. Obstet Gynecol. 2020;135(3):589-98.
4. Vargas MV, Cohen SL. Contained power morcellation: review of current evidence and techniques. Curr Opin Obstet Gynecol. 2019;31(4):246-52.
5. Yim GW, Kim SW, Nam EJ, Kim YT. Laparoscopic management of large adnexal masses using an endoscopic retrieval bag: oncologic safety and feasibility. Obstet Gynecol Sci. 2018;61(2):247-53.

12 CHAPTER

Techniques to Reduce Blood Loss in Laparoscopic Myomectomy

Mala Raj

ABSTRACT

Bleeding during myomectomy is the most common intraoperative challenge and a key determinant of operative morbidity, transfusion requirement, and conversion to laparotomy. Effective hemostasis combines pharmacologic, mechanical, and technical measures. Modern evidence supports the use of tranexamic acid, diluted vasopressin, temporary vascular occlusion, meticulous multilayer closure with barbed sutures, and adjunctive topical agents. This review discusses evidence-based strategies for securing hemostasis in laparoscopic myomectomy, focusing on safety, efficacy, and fertility preservation.

INTRODUCTION

Laparoscopic myomectomy has become a cornerstone procedure for women seeking uterine preservation in the management of symptomatic fibroids. Despite its advantages, intraoperative bleeding remains the principal concern. Excessive hemorrhage can prolong operative time, compromise visualization, and necessitate conversion to laparotomy. Therefore, developing a structured approach to hemostasis is critical. This article outlines a stepwise, evidence-based approach integrating preoperative, intraoperative, and postoperative strategies.

PREOPERATIVE OPTIMIZATION

Optimizing hemoglobin levels preoperatively is essential. Iron supplementation, erythropoietin therapy, and correction of coagulation disorders should be completed before surgery. Preoperative imaging, especially MRI or high-resolution ultrasound, delineates the vascular pattern and aids in planning incision sites and vascular control techniques.

PHARMACOLOGIC MEASURES

Tranexamic Acid

Tranexamic acid, an antifibrinolytic agent, stabilizes clot formation by inhibiting plasminogen activation. Several randomized controlled trials

(RCTs) and meta-analyses confirm its efficacy in reducing intraoperative blood loss and transfusion rates during myomectomy. A typical regimen involves administering 10 mg/kg (maximum 1 g) IV 10–15 minutes before incision. TXA is generally safe, though caution is advised in patients with a history of thrombosis.

Intramyometrial Vasopressin

Intramyometrial injection of diluted vasopressin produces local vasoconstriction and markedly reduces bleeding from myometrial sinuses. Evidence from systematic reviews supports its role in lowering blood loss and transfusion requirements. However, potential cardiovascular risks—bradycardia, hypertension, arrhythmias—necessitate strict dosing vigilance. Commonly, a 0.05–0.2 IU/mL dilution is used, and the total dose should not exceed 4–6 IU. Always aspirate before injection to avoid intravascular administration.

MECHANICAL AND VASCULAR CONTROL

Mechanical techniques aim to transiently reduce uterine perfusion during enucleation. Temporary uterine artery occlusion using clips, tourniquets, or vessel loops has proven effective in decreasing estimated blood loss. Several meta-analyses report significant reductions in blood loss and hemoglobin drop with these methods, especially in large or multiple fibroids. Care should be taken to limit occlusion duration to avoid ischemic damage. Preoperative uterine artery embolization (UAE) is another option for non-fertility-seeking women, but it is not routinely advised in fertility-preserving surgeries.

SURGICAL TECHNIQUE

Incision and Enucleation

A judiciously planned incision ensures minimal bleeding while preserving myometrial integrity. Sharp dissection with limited bipolar coagulation is preferred to avoid devascularization. Traction and counter-traction facilitate a clean cleavage plane.

Suturing and Closure

Meticulous multilayer closure of the myometrial defect restores uterine strength and ensures hemostasis. Barbed sutures, such as V-Loc or Stratafix, have demonstrated reduced suturing time and blood loss compared with conventional sutures in multiple RCTs and meta-analyses. Closure should proceed in two layers: deep myometrial approximation followed by serosal repair.

TOPICAL HEMOSTATIC AGENTS

When diffuse oozing persists after mechanical and pharmacologic measures, topical agents provide valuable adjunctive control. Agents like oxidized regenerated cellulose, fibrin sealants, and gelatin-thrombin matrices promote localized clotting and tissue adhesion. Their use should complement, not replace, proper suturing and surgical technique. According to ACOG guidelines, topical hemostats are appropriate for limited oozing in gynecologic surgery.

SUGGESTED INTRAOPERATIVE PROTOCOL

1. Preoperatively correct anemia and counsel the patient on blood-conservation strategies.
2. Administer tranexamic acid 10 mg/kg (max 1 g) IV 15 minutes before incision.
3. Inject diluted vasopressin (0.05–0.2 IU/mL) intramyometrially around the fibroid, aspirating before injection.
4. Apply temporary uterine artery occlusion or tourniquet for large/multiple fibroids.
5. Perform sharp dissection with minimal coagulation.
6. Suture in two layers using barbed sutures for deep and serosal closure.
7. Apply topical hemostats to residual oozing areas if needed.
8. Remove temporary occlusion and reassess hemostasis before closure.

DISCUSSION

Hemostasis during laparoscopic myomectomy determines not only operative safety but also long-term uterine integrity. The combination of systemic antifibrinolytics, local vasoconstrictors, mechanical occlusion, and refined suturing techniques minimizes bleeding. Barbed sutures, by maintaining consistent tension without knotting, have simplified layered closure. Temporary uterine artery occlusion remains particularly valuable for large or multiple fibroids but should be used judiciously in fertility-preserving cases.

Emerging evidence supports integrating multiple strategies rather than relying on a single measure. However, controversies remain—particularly around optimal vasopressin concentration, duration of vascular occlusion, and the fertility implications of temporary ischemia. Future RCTs should evaluate standardized hemostatic algorithms and long-term reproductive outcomes.

CONCLUSION

Securing hemostasis in laparoscopic myomectomy is a multifactorial process requiring preoperative optimization, pharmacologic adjuncts, and refined surgical technique. Tranexamic acid and diluted vasopressin significantly reduce intraoperative blood loss, while barbed sutures and temporary vascular occlusion enhance surgical efficiency. An individualized, evidence-based multimodal approach ensures safety, minimizes transfusion, and preserves fertility.

SUGGESTED READING

1. ACOG. ACOG Committee Opinion No. 812: Topical hemostatic agents in obstetrics and gynecology. Obstet Gynecol. 2020;136(4):e92-e101.
2. Angioli R. Use of temporary uterine artery occlusion in laparoscopic myomectomy: a systematic review and meta-analysis. J Minim Invasive Gynecol. 2020;27(1):50-8.
3. Kongnyuy EJ, Wiysonge CS. Interventions to reduce haemorrhage during myomectomy for fibroids. Cochrane Database Syst Rev. 2014;(8):CD005355.
4. Radosa MP. Laparoscopic myomectomy: impact of barbed versus conventional sutures on operative outcome. Fertil Steril. 2019;112(3):521-8.
5. Song T. The efficacy of tranexamic acid in reducing blood loss during laparoscopic myomectomy: A meta-analysis. Eur J Obstet Gynecol Reprod Biol. 2016;205:119-25.
6. Tinelli A. Vasopressin in laparoscopic myomectomy: safety and efficacy. J Minim Invasive Gynecol. 2017;24(2):192-8.

13 CHAPTER

Endometriosis and Pain Management

Prakash Trivedi, Aditi Trivedi, Soumil Trivedi

INTRODUCTION

Endometriosis perhaps is the disease of the millennium, a-sticky, perplexing and unconquerable pathology, remained an enigma and its etiology is not clearly defined, neither has a complete answer.

Our efforts in this text are to cover endometriosis and pain management.

INCIDENCE

Major issues are pain in abdomen, dysmenorrhea, dyspareunia, dyschezia, and pain at different sides of endometriosis. 65% pelvic pain/dysmenorrhea

Medical or laparoscopic surgery is one of the gold standards in treatment of endometrioma.

DEFINITION

Endometriosis is commonly defined as presence of endometrium at places other than the normal uterine cavity, invasive but non-neoplastic growth pattern.

Possible sites of endometriosis:

The disease may be limited more to the pelvis and lower abdominal organs plus beyond:

- Reproductive tract
- Urinary tract
- GI tract
- Surgical scars, umbilicus, episiotomy
- Lungs
- Rarely, pericardium, pleura, CNS, nose, eye

Susceptible tissues and organs are ovaries, uterosacral ligament, broad ligament, cardinal ligament, peritoneum of lower anterior abdominal wall, urinary bladder, round ligament, recto vaginal pouch, rectum, sigmoid colon, ureters, appendix, cecum, ascending colon, posterior vaginal fornix, vagina, peritoneum and site of episiotomy.

SYMPTOMS

The classical triad of dysmenorrhea, dyspareunia and infertility is the characteristic of the disease, the pain is often referred to rectum or lower sacral and coccygeal regions. Dysmenorrhea is progressive and not relieved by nonsteroidal anti-inflammatory drugs (NSAIDs). The symptoms are often cyclical meaning that the pain is worse right before or during the period and then improves.

Bowel and urinary problems including pain, diarrhea, constipation and bloating.

SIGNS

Bimanual pelvic examination may reveal tender uterosacral ligaments, cul de sac nodularity, induration of rectovaginal septum, fixed uterus, adnexal masses, generalized or localized pelvic tenderness.

DIAGNOSIS

Laparoscopy remains the gold standard in the diagnosis of endometriosis within the peritoneal cavity from the diaphragm to the pelvis.

But new imaging techniques have taken over in major endometriosis.

Ultrasound: Chocolate cyst of ovary as enlarged cyst with uniform granular hyperechoic fluid collection.

COLOR DOPPLER

It may demonstrate flow around but not within the endometriotic cyst.

Classical ultrasound findings are very useful but MRI is also complementary.

Endometriosis in teenagers, unmarried, they may be sexually active or not, history you have to take gently. Such females have symptoms of dysmenorrhea, severe pelvic pain, dyschezia or presence of 4–5 cm or more. The end points of treatment in such a group is absence of pain and improved quality of life. Laparoscopic surgery is best avoided as it can recur.

- 1st-line treatment was danazol but discontinued due to side effects, weight gain, hirsutism, cost, etc.
- 2nd COC's or only progesterone pills, but the issue is why give estrogen if endometriosis is estrogen dependent and why progesterone if it is not the cause of endometriosis. Progesterone only pill can counter estrogen effect.
- 3rd Dydrogesterone a retro progesterone does not suppress ovulation/ periods, yet have maximum concentration at endometriosis and

decidualize, also permits fertility. Can be used from day 5-25 or continuously. Pain score reduction and cost have to be compared.

- 4th GnRH depot 1 to 3 or 6 months leads to pseudomenopause may be taken for 3-6 months but thereafter add back therapy is needed like vitamin D, calcium, etc.
- 5th Dienogest effective for pain and can be used for long time especially if no interest in pregnancy
- 6th New oral GnRH antagonists hold promise for 3-6 months later and need add back therapy.

If endometrioma and pain is not reduced then laparoscopic surgery optimum by an expert should be done after checking AMH. The issue is 64% of endometriosis cases are treated by right or wrong method before 30-34 years of age.

Endometriosis or endometrioma during reproductive age group with or without pain

- The largest group of patients coming for treatment, hence it is most important to understand.
- Is the pain more important than infertility or vice versa?
- Extended medical treatment often deprives the fertility period of the patient.
- Further Per vaginal, bimanual examination, Per rectal exam, sonography and rarely MRI when essential.
- Large numbers of endometriomas if picked up early are not advanced diseases.
- They can be managed by laparoscopic surgery, dydrogesterone/short term oral GnRH antagonists and starting fertility treatment as the best immunological period for pregnancy is in 6-7 months after surgery.
- A standard ambulatory laparoscopic surgery followed by depo given by a gynecologist is not the best treatment.

The author has the largest experience of using dydrogesterone for 24 years postlaparoscopic surgery and starting ovulation induction drugs with or without IUI, planned relation or even IVF ICSI if needed, explained later. Short-term oral antagonists can be used in similar fashion esspecially if surgery was extensive or incomplete.

MANAGEMENT

Medical Therapy

In minimal to mild endometriosis: CPR were similar in the groups receiving GnRH-agonist treatment (6 months) or expectant management. Women treated with progestins or expectant management, pregnancy rates were similar.

GnRH Analogs

GnRH analogs in endometriosis are used in following conditions:

- Inflamed endometriosis or endometrioma
- Frozen pelvis or previous abdominal surgery for endometrioma
- Recurrent endometrioma treated by surgery
- Rectovaginal endometriosis or adenomyosis
- Postoperatively as a follow-up treatment to improve the pregnancy rates

In stimulation protocols for ART in patients with endometriosis of all grades

Advanced Endometriosis or with Rectovaginal Disease with or without Fertility

With the growth of excellent imaging experts and also abilities of laparoscopic surgeons to do extensive pelvic endometriosis rectovaginal, uterosacral ligaments has changed the situation globally. This entity has increased globally, with obvious over diagnosis.

Once you are at an endometriosis referral center, it goes without saying, after good imaging and good surgery pain relief is phenomenal when surgery is needed. Please note that such endometriosis does not respond to medical treatment and a surprise fair spontaneous pregnancy rate, plus on dydrogesterone treatment is noticed.

If patient's pain is more than fertility, please refer to laparoscopic expert on endometriosis advanced treatment.

UROGENITAL ENDOMETRIOSIS

Endometriosis of bladder, ureter, etc. comes with a unique blend, usually one cesarean section, no fertility issues. Further you can have cesarean scar endometriosis all excised by laparoscopic surgery and do not respond to medical treatment. Ureteric stent may be used no need of medical treatment postoperative and in due course of time they conceive if desired.

RECURRENT ENDOMETRIOSIS

- Endometriosis is a sticky disease and has recurrence rate of 25–75% irrespective of previous treatment.
- Management of recurrent endometriosis
- But if symptomatic usually it is with lots of adhesion around important structures. The laparoscopic surgery revolves around safety of surrounding structures ureter, bladder, bowels. Excision of optimum disease by an expert laparoscopist with a team is essential. Good post-operative care.

ENDOMETRIOSIS AT RARE SITES

- Episiotomy, port/cesarean scars, diaphragm, lungs and elsewhere. Essentially treatment of such disease is wide excision and no need of post-operative medicines except anti-inflammatory and serratiopeptidase to reduce inflammation and pain.
- Cesarean scar endometriosis is tricky as it has some rectal involvement. Proper laparoscopic excision. Closure of the defect and no medical treatment needed.
- Diaphragmatic endometriosis though rare needs laparoscopic excision and good suturing, if there is lung collapse then management is done with pulmonologist surgeon.
- *Localized adenomyoma:* Excision of adenomyoma—plane between normal myometrium and adenomyoma may be difficult to identify but is not a major concern. Closure is done by Vicryl or Barbed sutures or V Lock. Focal adenomyoma is better than diffuse involving the entire surface/wall. Difficulty in identifying plane. Vasopressin injection and planned incision, so that suturing of the defect can be done later-on. It may reach endometrial cavity.

Status of new oral GnRH antagonists: Benefits—

- Rapid onset of action compared to GnRH agonists.
- Avoidance of the initial estrogen "flare" seen with GnRH agonists.
- Effective in reducing pelvic pain, dysmenorrhea, and dyspareunia associated with endometriosis.
- Improves quality of life and reduces the need for surgical interventions.
- Endometriosis is a leading cause of infertility due to pelvic inflammation, altered ovarian function, and adhesions.
- Elagolix 150 mg or 200 mg twice daily had 50% to 32% ovulation. E2 dropped to 42 pg/mL at 150 mg and 12 pg/mL at 200 mg twice a day.
- Dysmenorrhea responder rates were reduced further by 7% in the 150 mg group and 17–18% on 6 months extension.
- For nonmenstrual pain 50.4%, 54.5%, 36.5% in respective group
- Elaris II had 49.8%, 57.8%, and 36.5% in respective groups
- Elagolix effectiveness in reducing endometriosis related pain on both bleeding and nonbleeding days providing consistent pain management throughout the cycle.

14 CHAPTER

Endometriosis and Fertility Optimization

Pandit Palaskar, Chintana Chandra

DEFINITION

Presence of endometrial like tissue (gland/stroma) outside the uterus.

Mainly associated with pelvic pain and infertility.

While 20–90% of women are symptomatic, 3–43% of women remain asymptomatic and 50% of women with or without pain present with unexplained infertility.

EPIDEMIOLOGY

Prevalence

- *Reproductive age group:* 10%
- Adolescents
- Postmenopausal women receiving HRT

Risk Factors

Association with ovarian cancer (endometrioid/clear cell): 1.3–1.9%

Protective Factors

See **Table 2**.

ETIOLOGY

Estrogen dependent states, explained by the following theories.

Theories

- Transplantation theory (by Sampson)
  In 70–90% women there is retrograde menstruation, i.e., seeding and implantation of endometriotic cells by trans tubal regurgitation of menstrual blood during menses into the dependent parts of pelvis.
- *Coelomic metaplasia:* Metaplasia of coelomic epithelium to endometrial tissue.
- *Induction theory:* Undefined biochemical factors induce undifferentiated peritoneal cells into endometrial tissue.

Factors Contributing to Endometriosis

- *Genetic:*
  - *Somatic mutation:* Plays role mostly in conversion to cancers.
  - *Germline mutation:* Risk of developing endometriosis increases *seven times* if first degree relative is affected.
- *Immunologic factors and inflammation:* Decreased immunologic clearance of viable endometrial cells from pelvic cavity during retrograde menstruation. Hence endometriosis is defined as "A state of subclinical peritoneal inflammation marked by increased peritoneal fluid volume, WBCs, cytokines, growth factors and angiogenesis promoting substances"
- *Environmental factors:* Dioxin and PCB exposure, but insufficient evidence.

CLINICAL FEATURES (TABLES 1 TO 3)

Site specific complaints like *cyclical* hemoptysis, hemothorax, dysuria, hematuria, pain abdomen depending on the affected organ.

Average delay in diagnosis: 3 years in patients with infertility and 6 years in patients with pelvic pain.

- *Pain:* Often bilateral and starts before the onset of menses, continues throughout the menses and persists after the elapse of menses (*triple dysmenorrhea*). Deep lesions present as pelvic pain and GI symptoms.

TABLE 1: Risk factors.

Early menarche	Red hair	LBW
Shorter cycle length	Tall height	One among twin
Nulliparity	Diet rich in red meat/fat	First degree affected relative
Hypermenorrhea	In utero DES exposure	Dioxin exposure
Infertility	Mullerian anomalies	Polychlorinated biphenyl exposure

TABLE 2: Protective factors.

Multiparity	High BMI
Lactation	High waist to hip ratio
Tobacco exposure in pregnancy	Diet rich in vegetarian

TABLE 3: Clinical features.

Dysmenorrhea	*GI symptoms:* Pain abdomen
Dyspareunia	Nausea and vomiting
Chronic pelvic pain	Bloating and early satiety
Infertility	Altered bowel habits, dyschezia

Mechanism:

- Local peritoneal inflammation
- Deep infiltration: Tissue damage
- Adhesions and Fibrosis: Distortion of normal anatomy and painful traction

- *Infertility:* 33% of infertile women are diagnosed with endometriosis whereas only 4% of fertile women are affected with endometriosis, suggesting direct correlation between infertility and endometriosis. Fertility improves in minimal to mild cases after surgical removal of endometriosis. Meanwhile in moderate to severe cases, due to adhesions there is reduced tubo-ovarian motility and low rates of successful ovum pick up affecting the fertility rates even after conservative surgeries.
- *Endocrine abnormalities:* Due to impaired follicular growth, there is decreased E2 levels during preovulatory phase and hence disturbed LH surge resulting in luteinized unruptured follicle syndrome and anovulation. Anovulation results in persistent rise in E2 (unopposed estrogen). Other conditions causing anovulation like hyperprolactinemia and hypothyroidism contribute similarly.
- *Extrapelvic endometriosis (1–2%):* Symptoms of pain or palpable mass occurring outside the pelvis in cyclic pattern.

DIAGNOSIS

Clinical Examination

- *Inspection:* vulva, vagina and cervix for visible lesions
- *Palpation:*

- Nodularity of POD/uterosacral
- Cervical displacement due to uterosacral scarring
- Tenderness in POD/cervical motion tenderness
- Ovarian cysts
- Fixed retroversion of uterus

Imaging

- *USG:* TVS—*"ground glass echogenicity of cyst fluid"*. Absence of findings on TVS does not rule out the presence of endometriosis, as it mainly subjective and depends more often on the quality of USG equipment **(Table 4)**.

TABLE 4: Sensitivity and specificity of TVS in endometrioma, DIE and peritoneal deposits.

TVS	*Endometrioma*	*DIE*	*Peritoneal deposits*
Sensitivity %	93	79	65
Specificity %	96	94	95

- *MRI:* Sensitive and specific for DIE and endometrioma, but expensive
- *CT:* Less role and unnecessary radiation exposure

Blood investigations: Raised CA125 in moderate-to-severe cases.

Gold standard: Laparoscopic visualization with histopathologic confirmation. Complete inspection and palpation with blunt probe for nodularity in the abdominal and pelvic cavity.

Laparoscopy findings:

- *Peritoneal endometriosis:* Typical *powder-burn* or *gunshot lesions* on the serosal surface of peritoneum, indicating old hemorrhage surrounded by fibrosis seen as black/dark brown/bluish cysts or nodules
- *DIE:* Lesions that are 5mm deep beneath the peritoneum presenting as nodules
- *Endometrioma:* Ovarian cysts also known as chocolate cysts containing thick viscous dark brown fluid composed of hemosiderin from previous hemorrhage.

  Histologic non affirmation does not exclude the disease.

*Laparoscopic classification **(Table 5)**:*

- *ASRM:* American Society for Reproductive Medicine Staging, most widely accepted surgical staging system **(Fig. 1)**.
- *ENZIAN:* To supplement ASRM staging with regard to the description of deep endometriosis, used in planning endometriosis surgery **(Fig. 3)**.
- *EFI:* Endometriosis Fertility Index, to predict non-IVF pregnancy rates for patients following surgical staging and treatment of endometriosis **(Fig. 2)**.

MANAGEMENT

Endometriosis is a chronic disease (30–60%) and recurrence rate is high even after both medical and surgical treatment.

- Treatment must be *individualized.*
- Taking into account clinical findings, impact of disease and effect of treatment on the quality of life.

TABLE 5: Various classification systems for endometriosis management and their utility.

ASRM	*ENZIAN*	*EFI*
For women undergoing surgery	DIE related staging	Prediction of natural pregnancy rate following conservative surgery
Based on appearance i.e., size, depth of peritoneal /& ovarian implants. Extent of adhesions and POD obliteration	ASRM staging+ site specific location and depth of DIE	Historical factors + ASRM staging+ functionality of tubes and ovaries

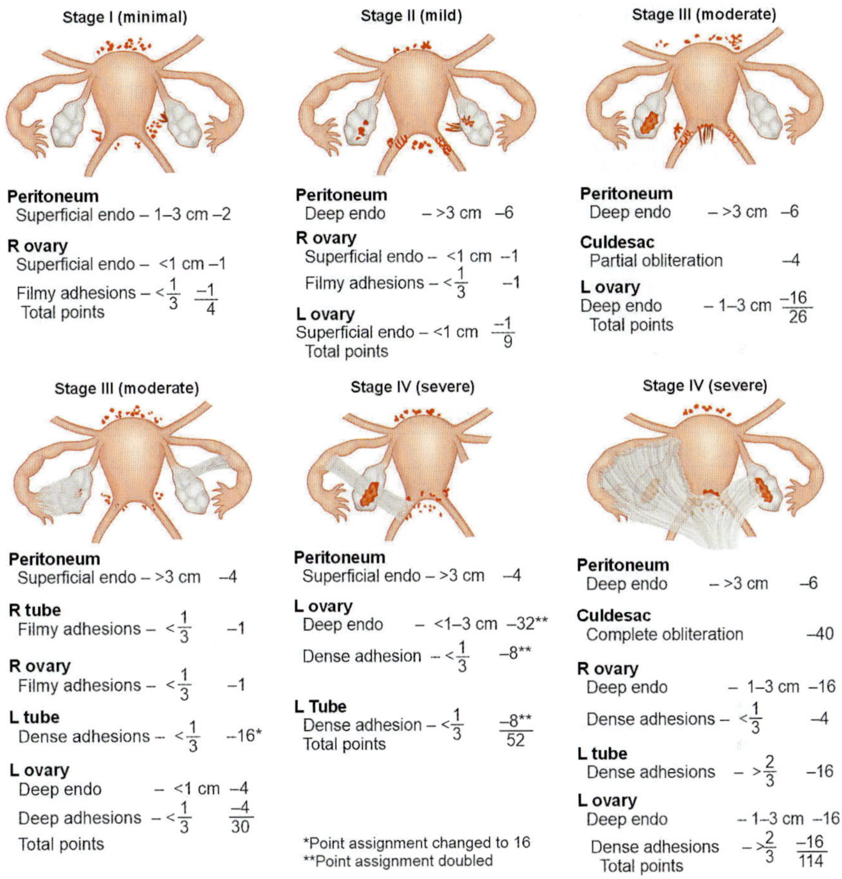

Fig. 1: ASRM staging.

- *Priority of patients:* Relief of pain/willingness for conception.
- Treatment of extragenital endometriosis (medical/surgical) depending on the site.

Medical Management of Pain

- *NSAIDs:* More effective than placebo for primary dysmenorrhea, but not so effective in endometriosis associated pain.
- *Hormonal treatment:* Pain relief is temporary as it resumes after cessation of medication. *Mechanism of action is mainly based on suppression of estrogen synthesis and induction of amenorrhea.*
    - *Oral contraceptive pills:* Use of cyclic OCPs provide prophylaxis against the development of recurrence of disease. Low dose monophasic OCPs containing ethinylestradiol of 20–35 mcg and norethisterone 1 mg/2.5 mg in OD dosage continuously or extended cyclic use for 6–12 months is safe and reduces dysmenorrhea, dyschezia, and deep dyspareunia significantly.

ENDOMETRIOSIS FERTILITY INDEX (EFI) SURGERY FORM

Least function (LF) score at *conclusion* of surgery

Score	Description		Left	Right
4 = Normal		Fallopian tube		
3 = Mild dysfunction				
2 = Moderate dysfunction		Fimbria		
1 = Severe dysfunction				
0 = Absent or nonfunctional		Ovary		

	Left		Right		LF score
Lowest score		+		=	

To calculate the LF score, add together the lowest score for the left side and the lowest score for the right side. If an ovary is absent on one side, the LF score is obtained by doubling the lowest score on the side with the ovary

ENDOMETRIOSIS FERTILITY INDEX (EFI)

Historical factors		Surgical factors	
Factor Description	**Points**	**Factor Description**	**Points**
Age		LF score	
If age is ≤35 years	2	If LF score = 7 to 8 (high score)	3
If age is 36 to 39 years	1	If LF score = 4 to 6 (moderate score)	2
If age is ≥40 years	0	If LF score = 1 to 3 (low score)	0
Years infertile		AFS endometriosis score	
If years infertile is ≤3	2	If AFS endometriosis lesion score is <16	1
If years infertile is >3	0	If AFS endometriosis lesion score is ≥ 6	0
Prior pregnancy		AFS total score	
If there is a history of a prior pregnancy	1	If AFS total score is <71	1
If there is no history of prior pregnancy	0	If AFS total score is ≥71	0
Total historical factors		Total surgical factors	

EFI = T total historical factors + total surgical factors:	Historical	+	Surgical	=	EFI score

Estimated percent pregnant by EFI score

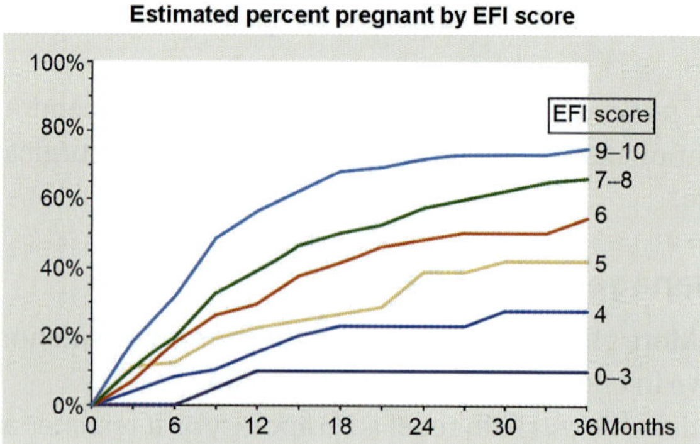

Fig. 2: Endometriosis fertility index (EFI).

- Vaginal ring containing 15 mcg of ethinylestradiol and 120 mcg of etonogestrel and transdermal patch containing 20 mcg of EE2 and 150 mcg of norelgestromin can be used, among which vaginal rings were more preferred.

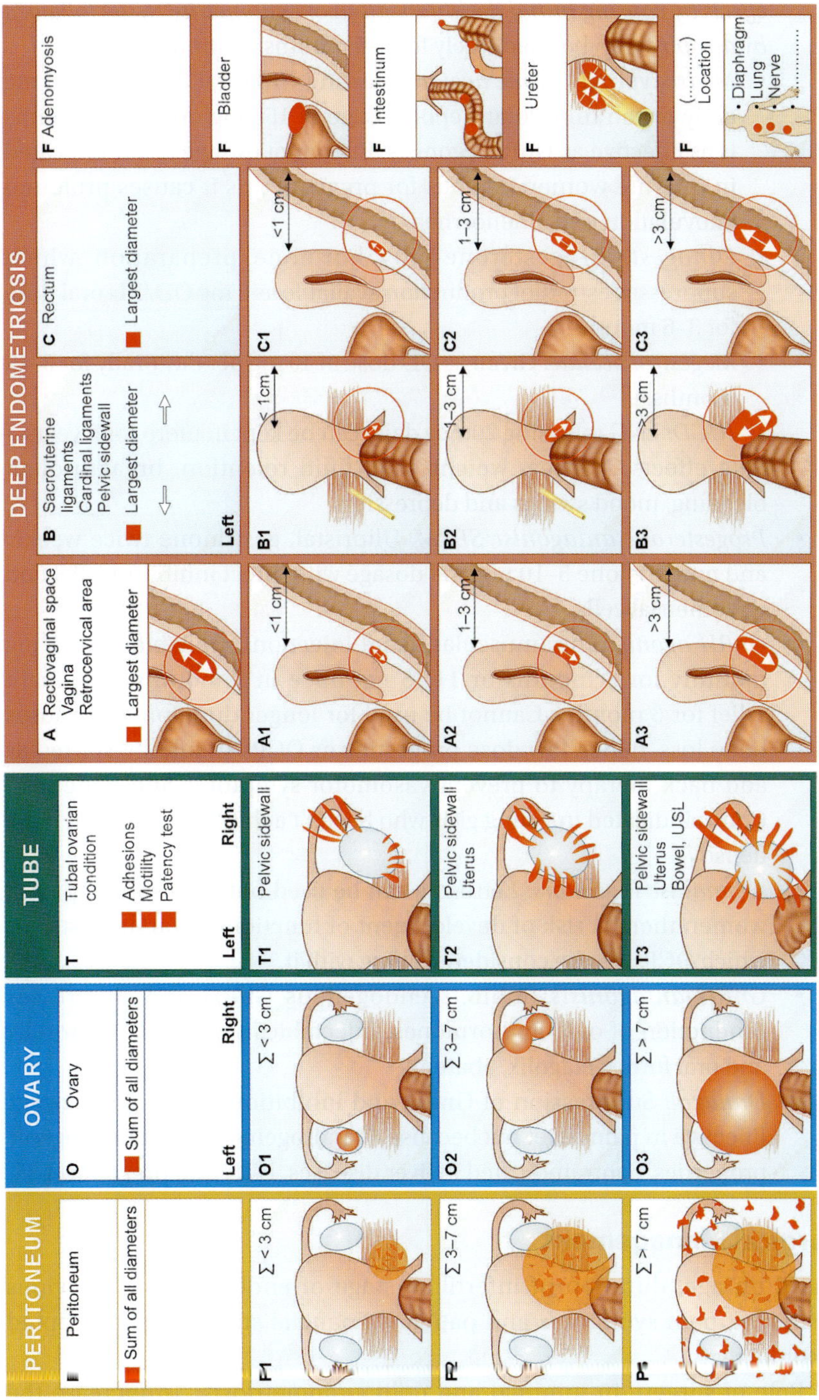

Fig. 3: ENZIAN Classification of endometriosis.

- *Progestins:* First choice of treatment as it *induces anti-endometriotic effects by causing initial decidualization of endometrial tissue followed by atrophy*. Can be used safely for 3–6 months continuously.
  - *Medroxyprogesterone acetate:* Starting with oral dosage of 30 mg daily or intramuscular depot dosage of 150 mg once in 3 months is as effective as GnRH agonists. But depot dosage is not indicated in infertile women anxious for pregnancy as it causes profound anovulation and amenorrhea.
  - *Dinogest:* Progesterone-only hormone preparation which suppresses estradiol production available as 2 mg OD/BD oral dose for 3–6 months.
  - *Megestrol acetate:* Given as OD dose of 40 mg per day orally for 6–12 months.
  - *IUCD:* LNG releasing 20mcg daily can be kept in utero for 5 years.

  Side effects: Nausea, weight gain, fluid retention, breakthrough bleeding, mood swings and depression.
- *Progesterone antagonist/SPRM:* Ulipristal, gestrinone twice weekly and mifepristone 5–10 mg oral dosage with direct inhibitory effect on endometrial cells.
- *GnRH agonist:* Intramuscular depot injections available as 3.75 mg monthly for 3 months or 11.75 mg once in 3 months gives pain relief for 6 months. Cannot be used for longer duration as it causes bone loss, hence low dose progestins or OCPs should be started as add back therapy to prevent vasomotor symptoms and bone loss. Contraindicated in young girls who haven't achieved maximum bone density.
- *Aromatase inhibitors:* Letrozole can be used but in postmenopausal women there is risk of development of functional ovarian cysts, for which OCPs can be considered along with it.
- *GnRH antagonists:* Inhibits endogenous GnRH and suppresses production of ovarian hormones. Injectables - ganirelix, cetrorelix and oral forms–elagolix, abarelix.
- *Danazol:* Suppression of GnRH and inhibition of steroidogenesis. Effective in pain relief but because of androgenic and hypoestrogenic properties, contraindicated in liver diseases, HTN and pregnancy.

Surgical Management

Based on age, duration of infertility, stage of endometriosis, previous treatment, pain symptoms and patients' financial state, surgery is opted accordingly.

- Role of surgery in minimal and mild endometriosis: To increase the chances of pregnancy.

- Role of surgery in moderate to severe endometriosis: To restore normal pelvic anatomy.

Motto: Excise all visible endometriotic lesions (peritoneal/ovarian cysts/DIE) and associated adhesions and restore normal pelvic anatomy.

Laparoscopy preferred over laparotomy due to quicker recovery, better cosmesis, less post operative pain and morbidity and fewer postoperative adhesions.

Conservative surgery:

1. Peritoneal endometriosis:
   - Excision
   - Bipolar coagulation
   - *Laser:* Carbon dioxide, potassium titanyl phosphate, argon laser
2. *Ovarian endometriosis:* ESHRE guideline recommends cystectomy over drainage and ablation as it has lower recurrence rate and better pain relief, although ovarian reserve is compromised in both treatments.
3. *DIE:* Complete surgical excision is preferred with due consents taken.

Nonetheless, there is negative correlation between stage of endometriosis and chances of natural pregnancy even after surgical removal of disease.

ESHRE guidelines for post operative hormonal therapy:

1. Females not seeking immediate conception after cystectomy for endometrioma.
2. As prophylaxis for endometriosis associated dysmenorrhea for at least 18-24 months.

Postoperative hormonal therapy is not routinely recommended because natural pregnancy rates during first 6–12 months after surgery is high. Nevertheless, it effective in reducing the recurrence rates and assuring better quality of life.

Management of Endometriosis in Adolescents

- *Common presentation:* Cyclic pain or chronic pelvic pain
- *Common stages:* Minimal-mild
- Medical management preferred initially; GnRH can be started only after 17 years of age.
- Laparoscopy should be considered in patients with chronic pelvic pain who do not respond to medical treatment as it 70% prevalent in such patients.

Management of Recurrent Endometriosis

Recurrence rate after cessation of medical treatment is almost 100% within 6–24 months and 2–20% per year after conservative surgery. It depends on the stage of disease, duration of follow up and completeness of previous surgery.

Prevention of recurrence: Plan pregnancy at the earliest, hormonal therapy until pregnancy and hysterectomy with bilateral oophorectomy in women over 40 years.

Role of ART

It is the only choice when tubo-ovarian anatomy is distorted and chances of natural pregnancy or follicular stimulation with intrauterine uterine insemination are reduced. After conservative surgery, 44% conceived naturally, 33% opted for ART by the end of 3 years among which 20% of them conceived through ART.

15 CHAPTER

Laparoscopic Burch Colposuspension: A Comprehensive Guide

Sejal Naik, Ritu Jain

INTRODUCTION

Laparoscopic Burch Colposuspension is a minimally invasive surgical technique designed to treat stress urinary incontinence (SUI) due to urethral hypermobility in women. Originally described as an open procedure by Dr John Burch in the 1960s, the laparoscopic adaptation maintains the same anatomical goals—elevating the bladder neck and proximal urethra to restore continence—while offering faster recovery and lower morbidity.

As awareness of mesh-related complications grows, non-mesh-based procedures like Burch Colposuspension are regaining popularity, especially among women seeking long-term solutions without synthetic materials.

ROLE IN THE MESH-FREE ERA

Considering growing concerns over synthetic mesh use, procedures like Burch Colposuspension offer effective, safe alternatives, particularly for young, active women or those with mesh complications.

Laparoscopic technique allows for enhanced recovery without compromising efficacy.

Note: Some studies suggest slightly lower long-term efficacy with laparoscopic approach, though outcomes are comparable in experienced hands.

INDICATIONS

Laparoscopic Burch is indicated in patients with:

- Genuine stress urinary incontinence (confirmed on urodynamics or clinical exam)
- Urethral hypermobility (Q-tip test >30°)
- Failed conservative management (pelvic floor physiotherapy, pessaries)
- Preference for non-mesh surgical options
- Patients undergoing laparoscopic hysterectomy or pelvic surgery—allowing combined procedures

TABLE 1: Contraindications.

Absolute	*Relative*
Active urinary tract infection	Dense pelvic adhesions
Intrinsic sphincter deficiency (ISD)	Previous failed continence surgeries
Poor surgical candidate (ASA IV/V)	Coexisting pelvic organ prolapses requiring another repair

CONTRAINDICATIONS

See **Table 1**.

PATIENT SELECTION AND COUNSELING

Ideal Candidates

- Women with confirmed urethral hypermobility and SUI
- Desire non-mesh surgical treatment
- No significant prolapse or ISD

Counseling Points

- Explain risks and success rates
- Compare with other options (TVT, TOT, slings)
- Stress on postoperative follow-up and bladder training

SURGICAL ANATOMY OVERVIEW

Space of Retzius: Retropubic area accessed during bladder dissection.

Cooper's ligament (pectineal ligament): Strong fibrous structure for anchoring sutures.

Endopelvic fascia: Tissue overlying the vaginal wall; site for suture placement near urethra/bladder neck.

The procedure targets the endopelvic fascia adjacent to the urethrovesical junction and bladder neck, suspending it bilaterally to the Cooper's ligament (iliopectineal ligament), creating a hammock-like support **(Fig. 1)**.

SURGICAL STEPS: LAPAROSCOPIC BURCH COLPOSUSPENSION (TABLE 2)

Preoperative Preparation

- Bladder catheterization
- Foley bulb inflated for bladder neck localization
- Prophylactic antibiotics

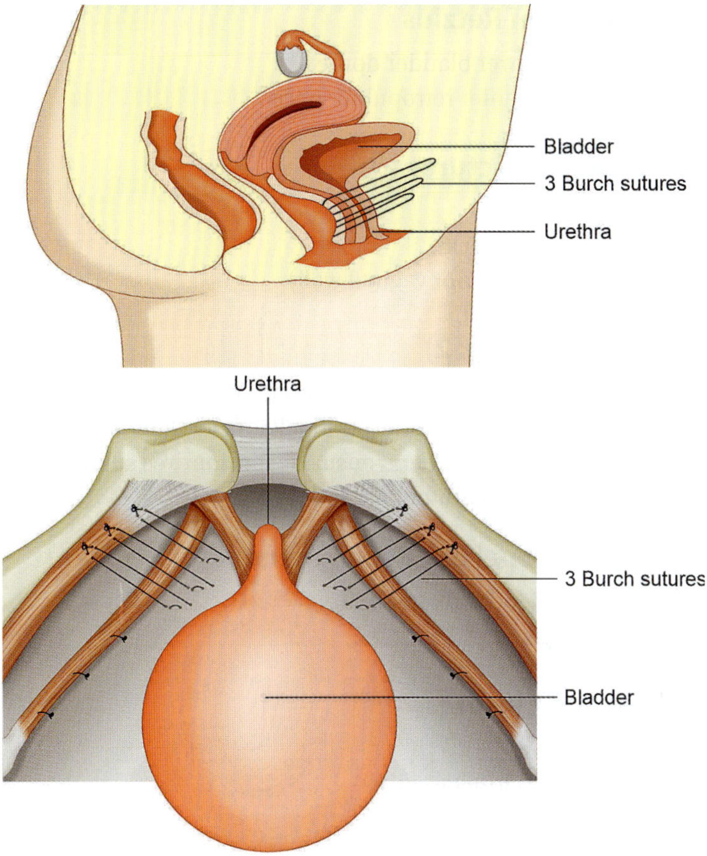

Fig. 1: Schematic representation of Burch's colposuspension.

TABLE 2: Key surgical points table.

Step	*Key tips*
Dissection	Stay midline to avoid vascular injury
Suture placement	1–1.5 cm lateral to urethra, avoid urethral penetration
Anchoring	Use strong bites in Cooper's ligament
Avoid overcorrection	Prevent bladder outlet obstruction
Check for bleeding/bladder injury	Use cystoscopy if in doubt

Positioning and Ports

- Lithotomy position with steep Trendelenburg
- 3–4 ports: One 10-mm umbilical camera port, Two or three 5-mm accessory ports in the lower quadrants

Accessing Space of Retzius

- Open peritoneum over bladder dome
- Blunt dissection to enter retropubic space

Identifying Key Structures

- Cooper's ligament
- Urethra and bladder neck
- Endopelvic fascia (anterior vaginal wall)

Suture Placement (Fig. 2)

- 2–3 non-absorbable sutures (e.g., Ethibond) placed on each side through the periurethral and paravaginal endopelvic fascia lateral to bladder neck
- Anchored to Cooper's ligament, ensuring tension-free support
- Avoid penetration into urethra or bladder

Cystoscopy (Optional but Recommended)

- Confirm no bladder or ureteral injury
- Check ureteric jets

Hemostasis and Closure

- Irrigation of space
- Remove ports and close fascia

Final Check

- Bladder integrity: Fill test
- Ureteric patency (optional)
- Secure hemostasis

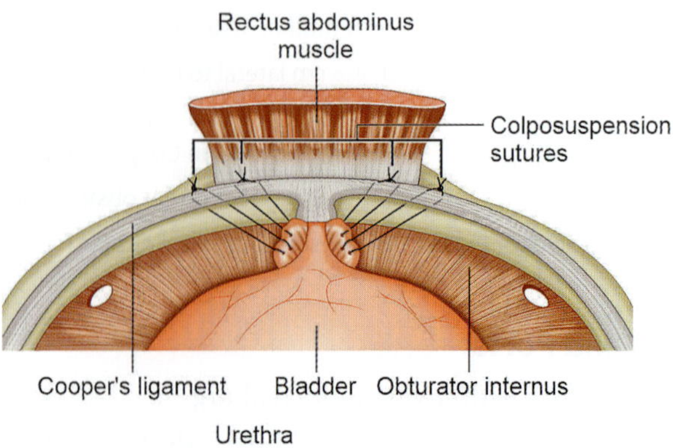

Fig. 2: Postcolposuspension picture.

POSTOPERATIVE CARE

- Catheterization: Foley for 24–48 hours
- Post-void residual check
- Voiding trial before discharge
- Analgesia and antibiotic prophylaxis
- Discharge typically day 1–2
- Resume normal activity in 2–3 weeks
- Avoid straining or heavy lifting for 4 weeks
- Monitor for urinary symptoms or retention
- Pelvic floor rehab recommended

ADVANTAGES OF LAPAROSCOPIC APPROACH (TABLE 3)

- Excellent visualization of anatomical landmarks
- Less blood loss
- Reduced postoperative pain
- Lower wound complications
- Shorter hospital stay
- Better cosmetic outcome
- Suitable for concurrent pelvic procedures

LIMITATIONS OF LAPAROSCOPIC APPROACH

- Requires advanced laparoscopic skills
- Longer operative time initially
- Lower success rate in certain high-risk patients

TABLE 3: Comparison: laparoscopic vs open burch procedure.

Parameter	*Laparoscopic Burch*	*Open Burch*
Invasiveness	Minimally invasive	Requires Pfannenstiel/lower midline
Hospital stay	1–2 days	3–5 days
Pain	Less	More postoperative pain
Recovery	Faster (2–3 weeks)	Longer (4–6 weeks)
Efficacy (5-year)	~80–85%	85–90%
Complications	Learning curve, possible bladder injury	Higher wound infection, longer stay
Cosmetic outcome	Better	Larger scar
Operative time	Slightly longer initially	Shorter for experienced hands
Visualization	Superior magnified view	Limited exposure

COMPARISON: LAPAROSCOPIC VERSUS OPEN BURCH

See **Table 3**.

ALTERNATIVE PROCEDURES FOR BURCH COLPOSUSPENSION

- Midurethral sling (MUS)—most used today, but involves mesh
- Autologous fascial sling—in cases with ISD
- Bulking agents—less invasive, but lower efficacy
- Conservative therapy—first-line for mild SUI
- Laser Therapy—Used in Mild SUI, though long term data lacking.

RECENT GUIDELINES AND EVIDENCE

- NICE (NG123)—Burch Colposuspension remains an option for women not suitable for synthetic mesh.
- ACOG Practice Bulletin 2015—Burch is effective and may be preferable in mesh-averse patients.
- Cochrane Review (2015)—No significant difference in long-term continence between laparoscopic and open Burch; laparoscopic has quicker recovery but longer operating time.

COMPLICATIONS

- Bladder or urethral injury
- Bleeding from venous plexus
- Urinary retention
- Overactive bladder symptoms
- De novo urgency or urge incontinence
- Voiding dysfunction
- Rarely: Wound or port-site complications

OUTCOMES AND SUCCESS RATES

- Reported success rates: 80–90% at 1–2 years
- Long-term success comparable to open Burch but may decline over time
- Effective in improving quality of life and continence
- Lower risk of complications vs mesh-based procedures

PRECAUTIONS DURING SURGERY

- Avoid over-elevation of bladder neck to prevent urinary retention
- Stay lateral to urethra while placing sutures
- Use gentle dissection in dense scarring
- Ensure Cooper's ligament is identified correctly to avoid vascular injury
- Prevent thermal injury from energy sources during dissection

- Avoid bladder perforation—confirm bladder boundary by preoperative backfill if needed

CONCLUSION

Laparoscopic Burch Colposuspension provides a safe, effective, and mesh-free option for treating stress urinary incontinence due to urethral hypermobility. Though technically demanding, its advantages in visualization, cosmesis, and recovery make it an attractive choice, especially in centers equipped for advanced laparoscopy.

Proper patient selection, surgical technique, and postoperative care are critical to achieving optimal outcomes. While open Burch remains the gold standard in long-term durability, laparoscopic Burch continues to evolve as a preferred option in minimally invasive urogynecology.

CHECKLIST: LAPAROSCOPIC BURCH COLPOSUSPENSION

Preoperative:
- Informed consent (non-mesh alternative)
- Urodynamic evaluation
- Rule out active UTI
- Bladder catheterization
- Prophylactic antibiotics

Intraoperative:
- Trendelenburg positioning
- Adequate exposure of Retzius space
- Identify bladder neck and Cooper's ligament
- Place 2 sutures on each side
- Anchor to Cooper's ligament (no tension)
- Avoid urethral/bladder injury
- Hemostasis check
- Bladder fill test

Postoperative:
- Foley catheter for 24–48 hours
- Voiding trial before discharge
- Watch for retention or urgency symptoms
- Advise pelvic rest 4–6 weeks

SUGGESTED READING

1. ACOG. ACOG Practice Bulletin No. 155: Urinary Incontinence. Obstet Gynecol. 2015;126(5):e66-e81.
2. Cochrane Review 2015: Open vs Laparoscopic Colposuspension.
3. Hilton P, Ward K. Efficacy of Burch Colposuspension at 5 years. Lancet. 1998.
4. P. Paraiso et al. Laparoscopic vs open Burch: long-term outcomes. Obstet Gynecol, 2002.
5. PM NICE NG123: Urinary Incontinence and Pelvic Organ Prolapse in Women, 2019.

2

SECTION

Hysteroscopy

16 CHAPTER

Hysteroscopic Evaluation of the Uterine Cavity

Vivek Marwah

INTRODUCTION

Hysteroscopy is a minimally invasive procedure used to directly visualize the interior of the uterine cavity. It allows real-time inspection of the endometrium, enabling precise diagnosis and targeted treatment. It is widely used in the evaluation of abnormal uterine bleeding (AUB), infertility, recurrent pregnancy loss, and suspected intrauterine abnormalities.

PRINCIPLES OF HYSTEROSCOPY

It involves the introduction of a hysteroscope—a slender telescope-like instrument—through the cervix into the uterine cavity. The hysteroscope is connected to a light source and camera, allowing visualization on a monitor. To improve visualization and access to intrauterine structures in the uterine cavity normal saline or glycine are usually used as a distension medium. The quality and resolution of the hysteroscopy visualization depends on the diameter of the hysteroscope used varying from 1.9 to 4 mm hysteroscopes.

INDICATIONS (TABLE 1)

Hysteroscopic evaluation is indicated in several clinical scenarios, including:

- Abnormal uterine bleeding (AUB).
- Subfertility and infertility work-up.
- Recurrent pregnancy loss.
- Suspected endometrial polyps or submucosal fibroids.
- Evaluation of uterine anomalies such as septate or bicornuate uterus.
- Removal of retained products of conception.
- Diagnosis and treatment of intrauterine adhesions (Asherman syndrome).
- Localization and removal of misplaced intrauterine devices (IUDs).

PREOPERATIVE CONSIDERATIONS

A thorough history and physical examination are essential. The procedure is typically performed in the early proliferative phase of the menstrual cycle when the endometrium is thin, aiding visualization. For postmenopausal assessment, it can be done anytime. Prophylactic antibiotics are not routinely

TABLE 1: Common abnormal findings.

Condition	*Hysteroscopic appearance*	*Clinical significance*
Endometrial Polyps	Smooth, pedunculated or sessile growths	May cause AUB or infertility
Submucosal Fibroids	Round, firm masses distorting cavity	Can impair implantation, cause bleeding
Endometrial Hyperplasia	Thickened, irregular endometrium	May indicate precancerous change
Intrauterine Adhesions (Asherman Syndrome)	Fibrous bands partially or fully obliterating cavity	Associated with infertility and menstrual abnormalities
Congenital Uterine Anomalies	Septum, bicornuate division, or irregular shape	Associated with pregnancy loss and infertility
Retained Products	Irregular vascular tissue remnants	Occur post-abortion or postpartum

needed unless there is a specific infection risk. Cervical priming using misoprostol may facilitate easier entry in nulliparous women or those with cervical stenosis.

Procedure Technique

- *Positioning:* The patient is placed in the lithotomy position.
- *Cervical Access:* After cleaning and draping, the cervix is stabilized. In office hysteroscopy, speculum insertion may be avoided by the "no-touch" vaginoscopic approach, reducing discomfort.
- *Introduction of the Hysteroscope:* The hysteroscope is gently passed through the cervical canal into the uterine cavity under direct visualization.
- *Cavity Observation:* The cavity is systematically examined:
  - Uterine fundus
  - Bilateral Ostia
  - Lateral walls
  - Anterior and posterior walls
  - Cervical canal on entry

Normal Findings

A normal uterine cavity appears triangular with smooth endometrial lining. The tubal ostia are seen as small dimples on the upper lateral corners.

ADVANTAGES OF HYSTEROSCOPY

- Accurate diagnosis.
- Option of diagnosis and treatment in one sitting.

- Minimally invasive
- Reduces need for hysterectomy in many cases.
- Decreases risks associated with blind procedures.

COMPLICATIONS

Though generally safe, complications can occur:

- *Uterine perforation:* May occur during cervical dilation or entry.
- *Bleeding:* Common during operative hysteroscopy.
- *Infection:* Rare but possible endometritis.
- *Fluid overload:* Excessive absorption of distension medium may lead to electrolyte imbalance or pulmonary edema.
  Careful monitoring and technique significantly reduce these risks.

POSTOPERATIVE CARE

Patients usually resume normal activities quickly. Mild cramping or spotting is common for 1–2 days. They are advised to report fever, heavy bleeding, or severe pain. If operative hysteroscopy was performed, additional follow-up may be required to monitor healing and treatment success.

ROLE IN MODERN GYNECOLOGY

Hysteroscopy has largely replaced blind D&C for diagnostic purposes. It plays a central role in infertility evaluation, especially in assisted reproductive techniques (ART), where even minor cavity abnormalities can influence implantation outcomes. Its ability to treat pathology at the same sitting makes it cost-effective and patient-friendly.

CONCLUSION

Hysteroscopic evaluation of the uterine cavity is a cornerstone in contemporary gynecological practice. Its minimally invasive nature, combined with the ability to directly visualize and manage intrauterine pathology, makes it invaluable in diagnosing and treating conditions related to abnormal bleeding, infertility, recurrent miscarriage, and intrauterine structural abnormalities. As techniques and technologies continue to improve, hysteroscopy will remain an essential, safe, and effective tool for uterine assessment.

KEY POINTS

- Hysteroscopy has largely replaced blind D&C for diagnostic purposes.
- Hysteroscopic evaluation of the uterine cavity is a cornerstone in contemporary gynecological practice.
- Its ability to treat pathology at the same sitting makes it cost-effective and patient-friendly.

- Its minimally invasive nature, combined with the ability to directly visualize and manage intrauterine pathology, makes it invaluable in diagnosing and treating conditions related to abnormal bleeding, infertility, recurrent miscarriage, and intrauterine structural abnormalities.
- As techniques and technologies continue to improve, hysteroscopy will remain an essential, safe, and effective tool for uterine assessment.

SUGGESTED READING

1. ACOG Committee Opinion No. 800 (March 2020): The Use of Hysteroscopy for the Diagnosis and Treatment of Intrauterine Pathology. HYPERLINK "https://www.acog.org/clinical/clinical-guidance/committee-opinion/articles/2020/03/the-use-of-hysteroscopy-for-the-diagnosis-and-treatment-of-intrauterine-pathology"ACOG Committee Opinion No. 800
2. ASRM Office Hysteroscopy Protocol: Office Hysteroscopy Procedural Guidance Source: American Society for Reproductive Medicine (ASRM) Highlights. HYPERLINK "https://connect.asrm.org/apppg/new-page/onboarding-resources/procedural-guidance-documents/office-hysteroscopy?ssopc=1"ASRM Office Hysteroscopy Guide
3. Cochrane Systematic Review: Hysteroscopy for treating subfertility and recurrent miscarriage Findings: Hysteroscopic treatment of intrauterine abnormalities improves reproductive outcomes in selected patients. HYPERLINK "https://www.cochranelibrary.com/"Cochrane Library – Hysteroscopy
4. ESHRE Guidelines: Management of Recurrent Pregnancy Loss (2023) Relevance. HYPERLINK "https://www.bing.com/search?q=%22https%3A%2F%2Fwww.eshre.eu%2FGuidelines-and-Legal%2FGuidelines%22"(eshre.eu in Bing)
5. FOGSI Good Clinical Practice Recommendations: Hysteroscopy in Infertility and AUB Highlights. HYPERLINK "https://www.fogsi.org/"https://www.fogsi.org
6. RCOG Green-top Guideline Update (September 2024): Outpatient Hysteroscopy – Updated Green-top Guideline. HYPERLINK "https://www.rcog.org.uk/news/rcog-publishes-update-to-green-top-guideline-on-outpatient-hysteroscopy/"RCOG Green-top Guideline.

17 CHAPTER

Hysteroscopy and Polypectomy: See and Treat

Venus Bansal, Ankita Sharma

INTRODUCTION

In the evaluation of intrauterine polyps the use of Hysteroscopy has become increasingly indispensable.

Polyps diagnosed by transvaginal ultrasound (TVUS) or MRI may still be missed or incompletely characterized. Even when a single polyp is visualized on imaging, hysteroscopy frequently reveals additional lesions, or shows the true extent of the polyp's base and its relations to the uterine wall, including near the cornu or internal os which may interfere with fertility. Moreover, the base of a polyp may harbor hyperplastic change or even malignant transformation that can be at times suspected during hysteroscopy, hence the base may carry a hidden cause of concern.

Hysteroscopy is a simple, low risk and cost effective outpatient procedure with an increased success rate.

Therefore, when intrauterine polyps are suspected—particularly in infertile women, in patients with abnormal uterine bleeding, or when imaging findings are equivocal—hysteroscopy not only secures diagnosis but enables simultaneous treatment. In essence: imaging suggests, hysteroscopy delivers.

In the chapter that follows, we will explore the indications, technique, operative considerations, and outcomes of hysteroscopic polypectomy, emphasizing why "see & treat" is the operative paradigm for uterine polyps.

INDICATIONS

The indications for hysteroscopic polypectomy according to recent guideline-level statements from the American College of Obstetricians and Gynecologists (ACOG) and the Royal College of Obstetricians and Gynaecologists (RCOG).

ACOG (USA)

From the ACOG Committee Opinion: "The Use of Hysteroscopy for the Diagnosis and Treatment of Intrauterine Pathology" (2020).

Key indications for polypectomy include:
- Abnormal uterine bleeding
- Infertility
- Recurrent pregnancy loss

The report also provides following general considerations:
- Direct visualization and removal of polyp to be preferred over blind techniques (blind curettage, blind polyp removal) because of superior accuracy and completeness.
- Office hysteroscopy for the treatment of endometrial polyps should be considered whenever possible
- Vaginoscopy may be considered while performing office hysteroscopy.

In summary, operative hysteroscopy (including polypectomy) is indicated when symptomatic or when there is likely benefit (e.g., bleeding, infertility, recurrent loss). The guideline does not state that every incidentally discovered asymptomatic polyp must always be removed — decision depends on symptoms, risk factors, fertility desires.

RCOG (UK)

From the RCOG "Outpatient Hysteroscopy (Green-top Guideline No. 59)" 2024. The guideline emphasizes that boundary between diagnostic and operative hysteroscopy is increasingly blurred (i.e., "see and treat" in outpatient setting) given advances in instrumentation. While it focuses more on the setting (outpatient vs theater) and patient experience, the implication is that operative hysteroscopy (including polypectomy) is appropriate when intrauterine lesions (such as polyps) are identified or strongly suspected and are contributing to symptoms or reproductive problems.

Indications for outpatient hysteroscopy:
- To aid the care of women/persons with abnormal uterine bleeding (including polyps).
- For the work-up of reproductive problems (infertility, recurrent miscarriage) when intrauterine pathology is suspected.

It recommends that vaginoscopy should be the standard technique for outpatient hysteroscopy and that mechanical hysteroscopic tissue removal system should be preferred over miniature bipolar electrode to remove endometrial polyps.

PRACTICAL CONSIDERATIONS

The decision to remove a polyp depends not just on its presence but on symptoms, fertility goals, risk factors for malignancy (e.g., post-menopausal status, tamoxifen use, bleeding) and technical feasibility. Blind curettage or blind removal is discouraged when accurate removal (and histology) is required—direct visual removal via hysteroscopy is preferred.

Appropriate patient selection for office based hysteroscopic procedures for women with known uterine pathology relies on thorough knowledge and understanding of the target pathology, size, depth and penetration of lesion, patients willingness to undergo the procedure, physicians skill and expertise, assessment of patient comorbidities and availability of proper equipment and patient support.

SCOPE SIZES, SHEATH DESIGN AND IMPLICATIONS

Modern diagnostic/operative hysteroscopes include very small diameters: For example, the Bettocchi continuous-flow operating hysteroscope comes in a 2.9 mm telescope with outer diameters of 4–5 mm when used with continuous flow and working channel. A larger operative scope might be in the 8 mm outer diameter or more.

The difference between a "small diagnostic/operative" scope (say ~2.9 mm telescope with ~4–5 mm sheath) and a larger operative scope (8 mm outer sheath) is important:

- Smaller scopes cause less cervical trauma, less need for dilation, allow potentially office setting use.
- Larger scopes allow bigger working channels, more robust instruments (loops, large bipolar electrodes), better irrigation/outflow, but require more dilation, possibly anesthesia and are generally OR-based.

Because flow and pressure dynamics differ with the internal volume of the sheath and the outflow channels, the same distension pump/setting designed for a larger scope may not give the correct pressure/flow for a smaller-diameter scope: the fluid volume, resistance, sheath cross-section, outflow fenestrations all affect intrauterine pressure, flow rate, turbulence and effectiveness of distension. A large sheath will allow higher flow for a given pressure while a small sheath may reach higher pressure or lower flow with same pump setting.

Therefore, when using a smaller scope, the infusion pressures/flow rates have to be lowered to avoid over-distending the uterus or forcing fluid through the tubal ostia into the peritoneum. Using the pump settings meant for larger sheaths on a small sheath, there will be risk of inaccurate reading of intrauterine pressure, excessive intrauterine pressure, fluid overload, or even mis-interpretation of vision because the outflow may be restricted causing higher pressure and reduced clearing of debris. ISGE recommends for diagnostic hysteroscopy pressures of <70 mm Hg (ideally 40–70 mm Hg) for small-diameter scopes to avoid spill into peritoneum.

Matching the hysteroscope sheath size + channel + inflow/outflow to the fluid/pressure system is essential, and the operator must be aware that "one size fits all" pump settings are *not* safe.

SPECIAL PRECAUTIONS SPECIFICALLY FOR POLYPECTOMY

- *Pre-procedure:* Ensure infection ruled out, informed consent obtained, discuss risks of fluid overload, perforation, bleeding, adhesion formation.
- Ensure the sheath tip is well-lubricated, warmed if needed, identify any cervical stenosis, dilate gently if needed.
- *For polyp removal operative cases:* After initial diagnostic survey you may switch to operative sheath/instruments—be aware of changing flow/resistance.
- *Distension fluid balance monitoring:* In operative cases you may have bleeding, irrigation fluid mixing with blood and saline—maintain accurate inflow/outflow chart to identify intravasation.
- *Visualization:* Clear view of polyp base before resection; be sure to define stalk, attachment, check adjacent endometrium.
- When removing polyps, ensure you take the entire base (include part of endometrium/myometrium if required) to reduce recurrence. Incomplete removal can lead to regrowth.
- Avoid excessive mechanical trauma to uterine wall; use gentle movements, maintain orientation to fundus/cornua.
- Avoid excessive intrauterine pressure, especially when using small diameter scopes or when bleeding is occurring (blood mixing reduces visibility). Keep pressure just enough to distend but not spill.
- When approaching polyp at internal os or near cornua, be careful about hitting tubal ostia or creating false passage, and always maintain visualization of instrument tip.
- *In infertile patients or when fertility preservation matters:* minimize thermal injury to endometrium/myometrium.
- *After removal:* Send specimen for histopathology; check cavity again for residual fragments; irrigate out debris; ensure outflow clearance.
- *Post-procedure:* Advise patient on mild cramping, spotting; restrict insertion (tampon/intercourse) as per protocol; monitor for fluid overload signs
- *Recognize and manage complications:*
  - *Peroperative:* Neurological and Compartment syndrome (proper positioning), General, Regional, local anesthesia (emphasis on vital monitoring and patients response)
  - *Intraoperative:* Cervical trauma, perforation uterus and adjacent organs (stop immediately), Distension media and fluid overload/hyponatremia (monitor volumes), Gas embolism, Perforation-, Bleeding-cervical and uterine (compress or insert balloon if, needed), pelvic vessels (immediate laparotomy), Electrosurgical-local, remote (immediate laparotomy)

- *Postoperative Infection:* Endomyometritis, peritonitis, Asherman's, Pregnancy related—uterine rupture, placenta accreta, increta

INSTRUMENTATION EVOLUTION AND RETRIEVAL TECHNIQUE

Historical to Current Progression

- *Monopolar resection loops:* In older operative hysteroscopy, removal of polyps/myomas was done using monopolar loops requiring non-conductive distension media (e.g., 1.5% glycine) and generation of thermal energy. Disadvantages: Risk of fluid absorption, hyponatremia, thermal damage to adjacent endometrium/myometrium.
- *Bipolar resection electrodes:* More recent shift to bipolar systems allows use of isotonic saline, less risk of hyponatremia, less thermal spread, improved safety, faster recovery. Example: mini bipolar 5 Fr electrodes for office hysteroscopy.
- *Mechanical tissue shavers ("morcellator"/tissue removal devices):* The latest generation - a small tip (~5.3 mm) with cutting window, suction, and blade that shaves tissue while aspirating the chips. This mechanical removal is especially useful for polyps and small fibroids in office or OR setting, with minimal thermal injury.
- *Cold scissors/graspers (5 Fr instruments through small sheaths):* Especially in office setting you can use 5 Fr scissors/forceps through continuous-flow small diameter scopes to remove small polyps without any energy. Advantages: minimal thermal injury, fertility-friendly, low cost, minimal fluid usage.

Instrument Choice and Retrieval Technique

- *For small polyps (especially office setting):* Use small diameter continuous-flow hysteroscope (2.9 mm telescope + ~4 mm sheath) with 5 Fr grasping forceps or scissors to remove polyp; retrieve with forceps or small basket; minimal dilation required. Using scissors had low recurrence compared to graspers.
- *For larger polyps, or if multiple polyps or broader base:* Use operative sheath (5 mm or larger), possibly tissue shaver, bipolar loop or morcellator.
- After cutting/removing the polyp, always inspect the base, possibly coagulate the base slightly (if thermal device used) or shave remaining tissue mechanically to reduce recurrence.
- *Retrieve specimen completely:* ensure no residual fragments remain. Use suction or irrigation to flush debris.
- When using mechanical shaver, you have simultaneous cutting + aspiration which reduces time and fluid usage.

- *For retrieval limitations:* small working channel (5 Fr) may limit the size of instrument and retrieval bag; for larger lesions you may need resectoscope or dump retrieval bag.
- *Post-removal inspection:* ensure tubal ostia, cornua, fundus and walls are clear; switch back to diagnostic sheath if you used larger sheath to allow clearer view of cavity.

SUMMARY OF KEY POINTERS

- *Choose appropriate hysteroscope size:* smaller for simple polyp removal (2.9 mm telescope + 4–5 mm sheath) and larger for extensive operative work.
- *Adjust fluid/pressure settings according to sheath size:* for small scopes keep pressure ~40–70 mmHg and monitor flow; don't use settings meant for large scope blindly.
- Use vaginoscopic/no-touch approach (Bettocchi) when feasible for patient comfort.
- Visualize cervix, internal os, cornua carefully before operating—especially important when polyps may be near internal os or cornu.
- *Select instruments:* mechanical scissors, forceps, bipolar loop or shaver.
- Ensure minimal thermal damage to the endometrium.
- Retrieve all tissue, inspect base, flush debris.
- Monitor fluid balance, avoid excessive intrauterine pressure, manage complications.
- The evolution from monopolar → bipolar → mechanical shaver/cold instruments has significantly improved safety, fertility outcomes, patient comfort and recovery.

SUGGESTED READING

1. ACOG. The Use of Hysteroscopy for the Diagnosis and Treatment of Intrauterine Pathology: ACOG Committee Opinion, Number 800. Obstet Gynecol. 2020;135(3):e138-e48.
2. De Silva PM, Smith PP, Cooper NA, Clark TJ. Outpatient hysteroscopy: (Green-top guideline no. 59). BJOG. 2024;131:e86-e110.
3. De Vree B. Diagnostic Hysteroscopy: equipment and technique. Trocar. 2023;4(1):12-22.
4. Hashemi M, Madani ES, Ghahiri A, Tarrahi MJ, Rouholamin S. Assessment of Long- and Short-Term Outcomes of Hysteroscopic Polypectomy in Patients with Uterine Polyps. Adv Biomed Res. 2024;13:57.
5. Triantafyllidou O, Korompokis I, Chasiakou S, Bakas P, Kalampokas T, Simopoulou M, et al. Impact of Hysteroscopic Polypectomy on IVF Outcomes in Women with Unexplained Infertility. J Clin Med. 2024;13(16):4755.
6. Vitale SG, Haimovich S, Laganà AS, Alonso L, Di Spiezio Sardo A, Carugno J, et al. Endometrial polyps. An evidence-based diagnosis and management guide. Eur J Obstet Gynecol Reprod Biol. 2021;260:70-7.

18 CHAPTER

Tubal Cannulation

Ajay Aggarwal, Aarti Chitkara Wadhawan

INTRODUCTION

Tubal factor infertility continues to be one of the leading contributors to female infertility, accounting for nearly one-quarter to one-third of all cases. Within this category, proximal tubal obstruction constitutes 10 to 25% of tubal pathology and is a frequent cause of infertility requiring targeted intervention. The history of proximal tubal surgery reflects significant innovation. In 1977, selective transcervical tubal cannulation was first described using a Grafia catheter to introduce contrast medium into the tubal lumen. This foundational step paved the way for more advanced procedures. A major milestone was reached in 1988 when Novy et al. performed the first hysteroscopic cannulation under laparoscopic guidance. Over subsequent decades, improvements in imaging, catheter design, and operative hysteroscopy have made fluoroscopy-guided and hysteroscopy-guided selective salpingography standard techniques in modern practice.

The role of tubal surgery, however, continues to be evaluated in the broader context of assisted reproductive technology. IVF offers high per-cycle success rates and bypasses tubal pathology entirely, yet tubal surgery—including tubal cannulation—remains relevant for selected women. The decision between IVF and corrective tubal surgery requires individualized assessment, shared decision-making, and thorough patient counseling. Factors such as the woman's age, ovarian reserve, tubal anatomy, surgeon expertise, cost considerations, and reproductive goals all influence the final choice. Tubal cannulation, especially, is attractive because it is minimally invasive, has a high success rate in nonfibrotic proximal disease, and allows natural conception.

DIAGNOSIS

A structured diagnostic approach is essential to identify the underlying cause and extent of tubal disease. The initial evaluation begins with a detailed medical, surgical, and reproductive history. Important clues include a history of pelvic inflammatory disease, previous ectopic pregnancy, sexually transmitted infections, tuberculosis, endometriosis or pelvic surgeries such as myomectomy or cystectomy. Many of these conditions may cause tubal inflammation, scarring, or blockage.

Hysterosalpingography (HSG) remains the first-line investigation for evaluating tubal patency. Its widespread use is due to accessibility, cost-effectiveness, and ability to provide both diagnostic and sometimes therapeutic benefits. HSG has a sensitivity of nearly 89% but a lower specificity of around 45%, largely due to false-positive findings resulting from temporary tubal spasm or inadequate contrast flow. Despite these limitations, HSG can improve fertility outcomes through the "tubal flushing effect," particularly when oil-based contrast agents are used, which may remove debris or mucus plugs.

In cases where HSG suggests proximal obstruction, further confirmation is recommended before proceeding with surgery. Options include repeat HSG, saline infusion sonography with contrast (HyCoSy) and hysteroscopy. This step helps distinguish true anatomic obstruction from transient spasm and prevents unnecessary intervention.

PREOPERATIVE CONSIDERATIONS

Choosing between tubal surgery and IVF requires thoughtful consideration of medical, reproductive, and psychosocial factors. Key elements include:

- *Age of the woman:* Fertility declines significantly after age 35, making IVF more appealing in older women.
- *Ovarian reserve:* Poor ovarian reserve may favor IVF to maximize time-sensitive fertility potential.
- *Prior fertility and reproductive intentions:* Women desiring multiple children may benefit more from tubal surgery.
- *Tubal disease severity:* Mild proximal obstruction favors cannulation; severe distal disease may require IVF.
- *Presence of male factor infertility:* Significant abnormalities in semen parameters shift management toward IVF.
- *Other infertility factors:* Anovulation, diminished reserve, severe endometriosis, or uterine anomalies influence decision-making.
- *Cost and reimbursement:* IVF can be expensive; tubal surgery is often more affordable.
- *Religious, cultural, and personal beliefs:* Some couples prefer natural conception.
- *Surgeon skill and experience:* Outcomes improve in centers with expertise in tubal microsurgery or hysteroscopic cannulation.
- *Local IVF success rates:* Wide variability exists between clinics.

During counseling, the advantages and disadvantages of both options should be clearly presented. IVF has a high per-cycle success rate, avoids tubal surgery and bypasses tubal damage, but requires multiple injections, monitoring, and carries risks such as ovarian hyperstimulation syndrome and multiple pregnancy. Tubal surgery, conversely, allows for spontaneous conception every cycle, avoids the medical burden of IVF and can result in multiple future pregnancies without repeat intervention, though outcomes depend heavily on the underlying condition of the tubes and surgical expertise.

PREOPERATIVE EVALUATION

A complete assessment is essential before proceeding with tubal cannulation. The recommended evaluation includes:

- *Routine investigations:* Complete blood count, coagulation profile, renal and liver function tests, and virology screening.
- *Endocrine assessment:* Thyroid-stimulating hormone (TSH), anti-Müllerian hormone (AMH), day-2/3 FSH and LH, and mid-luteal progesterone.
- *Pelvic ultrasonography:* Evaluation for ovarian reserve, uterine pathology, hydrosalpinx, or adhesions.
- *Hysterosalpingography:* Assessment of uterine cavity and tubal patency.
- *Semen analysis:* Mandatory evaluation for all male partners.

This comprehensive approach ensures that the patient is appropriately selected and optimally prepared for surgery.

CONTRAINDICATIONS

Tubal cannulation is not appropriate in the following situations:

- Active pelvic infection or genital tuberculosis
- Tubal block at multiple anatomical levels
- Extensive tubal damage or previous failed tubal surgery
- Severe male factor infertility where IVF provides better outcomes
- Hydrosalpinx requiring salpingectomy prior to IVF

PROCEDURE FOR PROXIMAL TUBAL BLOCKAGE

Proximal tubal obstruction may arise from functional causes such as tubal spasm or mucus plugs, or from anatomical causes including fibrosis and scarring and accounts for 10–25% of tubal disease. Functional causes are highly amenable to cannulation, whereas true anatomical obstruction due to salpingitis isthmica nodosa, chronic infection, or endometriosis requires more complex management.

Before proceeding with proximal cannulation, it is essential to document normal distal tubal anatomy. Laparoscopy or ultrasonography can evaluate fimbrial morphology, tubal caliber, and pelvic adhesions. Success of proximal repair depends heavily on distal tubal integrity.

Modern approaches to cannulation include:

- Hysteroscopy-guided cannulation under laparoscopic visualization
- Fluoroscopy-guided selective salpingography

- Coaxial catheter systems
- Ultrasound-guided transcervical cannulation
- Falloposcopy (less commonly used)

The coaxial system typically includes an outer catheter positioned at the uterotubal ostium and an inner flexible guidewire used to traverse the occlusion. Under fluoroscopy, selective salpingography can assess tubal patency before and after recanalization.

Failure to pass the guidewire despite gentle pressure indicates true anatomical obstruction, at which point the procedure is terminated to prevent perforation. In these women, IVF is generally recommended. However, in those who decline IVF, surgical resection and microsurgical anastomosis may be considered.

Despite successful cannulation, approximately one-third of tubes may re-occlude. Perforation rates range from 3 to 11%, although most cases have no major clinical consequences.

A recent meta-analysis suggests pooled pregnancy rates of 31% for the hysteroscopic approach of tubal cannulation. Laparoscopy also offers the advantage of assessing additional pelvic factors, including distal tubal status and the tubo-ovarian relationship.

LAPAROSCOPIC-GUIDED HYSTEROSCOPIC TUBAL CANNULATION

The procedure is usually performed in the early proliferative phase when the endometrium is thin and visibility optimal.

Laparoscopy

Laparoscopy begins with a thorough survey of pelvic anatomy, including the uterus, ovaries, and fallopian tubes. Adhesions, endometriosis, or pelvic pathology are documented. A methylene blue dye test is performed to confirm proximal obstruction. Lack of spill from the affected tube supports the diagnosis and allows progression to hysteroscopic cannulation.

Hysteroscopy

A 5-mm hysteroscope is introduced through the cervix. The uterine cavity and both tubal ostia are visualized. A 5 Fr cannulation set is passed through the operative channel or alongside the hysteroscope **(Figs. 1A and 1B)**. Under direct vision, the catheter is aligned with the affected ostium and the stent is gently advanced 3 to 4 mm into the proximal tubal lumen **(Figs. 2A and B)**. Correct placement is confirmed laparoscopically, ensuring no perforation has occurred **(Fig. 3)**. Under laparoscopic visualization, the stent is advanced further into the tubal lumen to confirm free mobility. The catheter is then advanced over the stent and positioned securely at the tubal

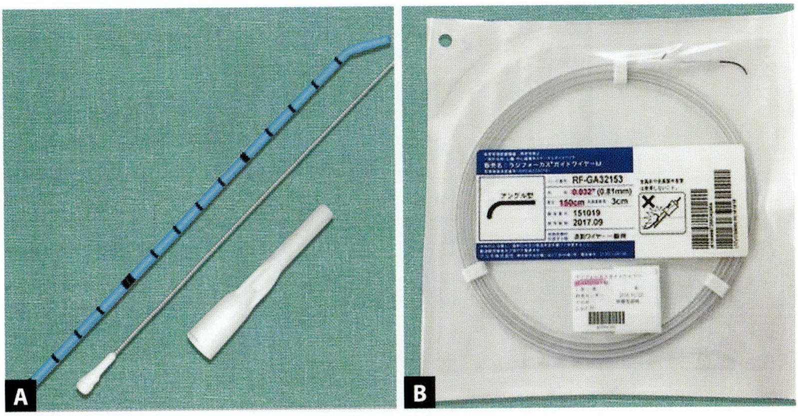

Figs. 1A and B: (A) Ureteric catheter; (B) Flexible guidewire.

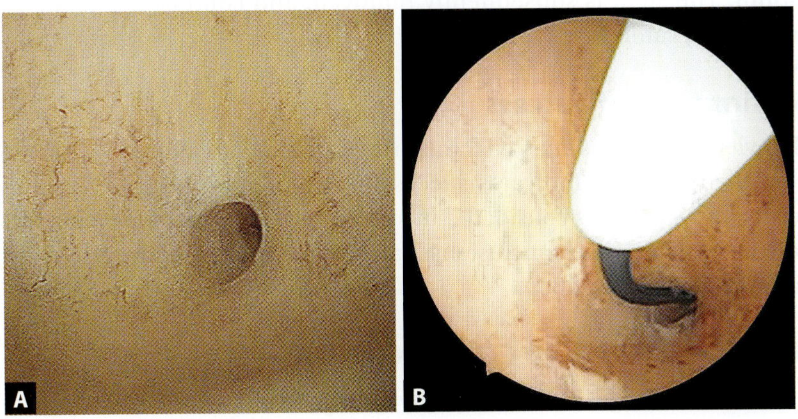

Figs. 2A and B: Tubal ostium before and after cannulation.

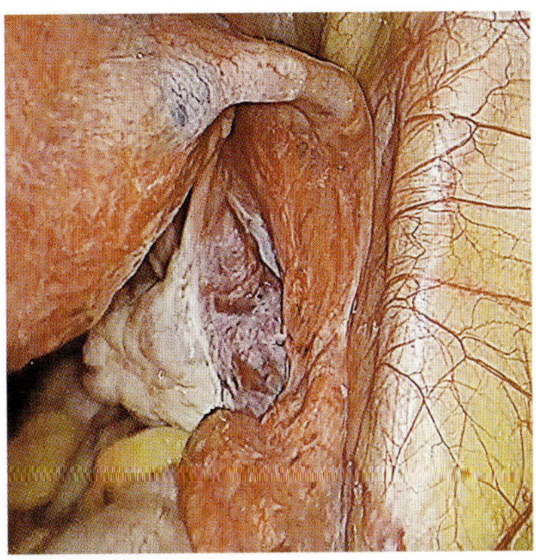

Fig. 3: Laparoscopic confirmation of guidewire in the proximal tube.

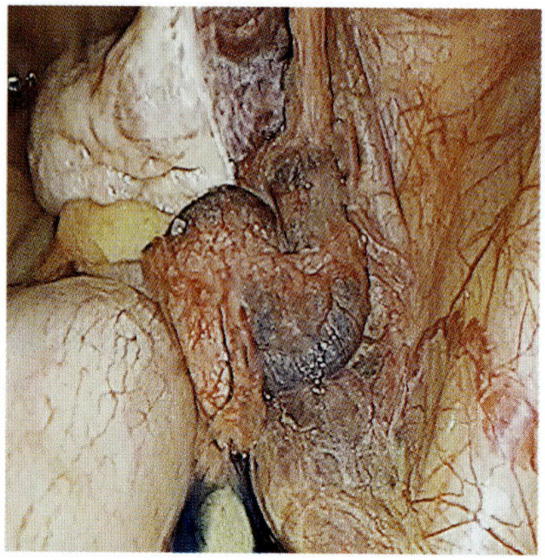

Fig. 4: Free spill of dye through distal end.

ostium. The stent is subsequently removed, and contrast dye is injected through the catheter.

Confirmation of Success

Methylene blue dye is injected through the cannulation catheter. Free spillage from the distal end indicates successful cannulation **(Fig. 4)**. If no spill occurs, the attempt is considered unsuccessful. Observing the contralateral tube helps avoid false conclusions, particularly in cases of dye backflow or pressure misinterpretation.

DIFFICULTIES AND COMPLICATIONS

Technical challenges include inability to negotiate the obstruction, mucosal edema from prolonged manipulation, kinking of the catheter, or poor visualization in cases of Asherman syndrome. Complications may include partial tubal perforation at the cornual end, intravasation of methylene blue into uterine vessels, persistent obstruction, ectopic pregnancy, infection, and bleeding.

SUMMARY

Effective management of tubal infertility requires a comprehensive understanding of the patient's clinical profile, reproductive goals, tubal pathology, and available resources. Although IVF provides high per-cycle success rates, tubal surgery—and tubal cannulation in particular—offers a minimally invasive, cost-effective alternative for women with correctable proximal obstruction. With proper patient selection, hysteroscopic or fluoroscopic tubal cannulation yields excellent outcomes and allows natural conception, making it a valuable component of modern infertility management.

SUGGESTED READING

1. ACOG. Infertility workup for the women's health specialist: ACOG committee opinion, number 781. Obstet Gynecol. 2019;133:e377-84.
2. De Silva PM, Chu JJ, Gallos ID, Vidyasagar AT, Robinson L, Coomarasamy A. Fallopian tube catheterization in the treatment of proximal tubal obstruction: a systematic review and meta-analysis. Hum Reprod. 2017;32:836-52.
3. Honore GM, Holden AE, Schenken RS. Pathophysiology and management of proximal tubal blockage. Fertil Steril. 1999;71:785-95.
4. Mohiyiddeen L, Hardiman A, Fitzgerald C, Hughes E, Mol BW, Johnson N, et al. Tubal flushing for subfertility. Cochrane Database Syst Rev. 2015;2015(5):CD003718.
5. Pinto AB, Hovsepian DM, Wattanakumtornkul S, Pilgram TK. Pregnancy outcomes after fallopian tube recanalization: oil-based versus water-soluble contrast agents. J Vasc Interv Radiol. 2003;14(1):69-74.

19 CHAPTER

Septum Resection

Soumil Trivedi, Kaustav Kar

INTRODUCTION

A uterine septum is the most common Müllerian anomaly encountered in gynecology and remains a frequent target for hysteroscopic surgery. Over the last decade, practice has shifted from routine resection of any septum to a more nuanced, evidence-informed, patient-centered approach. This chapter entails current classification, indications, operative options, perioperative techniques to improve safety and fertility outcomes, and recent innovations that are changing how hysteroscopic septum resection is performed.

ANATOMY, EMBRYOLOGY, AND DEFINITIONS

A septate uterus arises from incomplete resorption of the midline Müllerian ridge. Modern diagnostic criteria vary: the 2021 ASRM update and competing ESHRE-ESGE/CUME criteria differ in cut-offs for indentation depth and angle; this variability affects prevalence estimates and decision-making.

Practically, many now adopt the 2021 ASRM criteria (endometrial septum length >10 mm with indentation angle <90°) when deciding management pathways. Correct classification is crucial because it underpins indications for intervention.

INDICATIONS AND PATIENT SELECTION

Historically, septum resection was recommended for women with recurrent miscarriage, infertility or adverse obstetric history. However, high-quality evidence has produced conflicting outcomes.

- A large randomized trial (Rikken et al., 2021) reported *no overall reproductive benefit* to septum resection versus expectant management, creating controversy.
- Several systematic reviews/meta-analyses report possible improvements in selected subgroups—recurrent pregnancy loss, infertility—but evidence quality varies.

Current guideline thinking emphasizes *shared decision-making*, especially in recurrent miscarriage and before ART.

The most recent *ASRM Practice Guidance (2024)* recommends individualized counseling rather than blanket resection of all septa.

PREOPERATIVE ASSESSMENT AND PLANNING

- *Imaging:* 3D-TVUS is the preferred diagnostic tool for defining cavity shape and septal characteristics. Saline-infusion sonography and MRI are used as adjuncts specially in aberrant anatomy.
- *Counseling:* Discuss fertility prognosis, risks (perforation, bleeding, fluid overload, hyponatremia, adhesions), possible need for staged procedures, and alternatives (expectant management). For patients undergoing ART, discuss timing relative to IVF cycles.

OPERATING THEATER VERSUS OFFICE SETTING

Office hysteroscopy and ambulatory surgery are increasingly used for small-to-moderate septa. Advances in mini-hysteroscopes (3–5 mm), 5-Fr instruments and vaginoscopic techniques permit office resection for thin or moderate septa.

However, longer or thick septa, suspected myometrial involvement, or concomitant intracavitary pathology may still require an operating theatre and general or regional anesthesia. Office hysteroscopy is safe, effective and patient-preferred when appropriately selected.

SURGICAL TECHNIQUES—PRACTICAL APPROACH

Mechanical (Scissors) Technique

Hysteroscopic scissors (rigid or semi-rigid 5-Fr) or cold knife via mini-hysteroscope allow precise, tissue-sparing incisions with no electrosurgery. Advantages include low thermal damage, better fertility outcome and ease in office setting; however, hemostasis may be less straightforward for bleeding septa. Modern 5-Fr instruments facilitate office management.

Electrosurgical Resection

Traditional resectoscopes (15–26 Fr) with monopolar loop have been used for decades. Bipolar systems (using saline as distension medium) reduce the risk of hyponatremia, glycine toxicity and may have improved fluid safety profiles; comparative studies suggest similar reproductive and operative outcomes but improved fluid management with bipolar energy. Careful stepwise resection to the level of normal endometrium with intraoperative landmarks avoids over-resection.

Lasers

The use of hysteroscopic lasers, particularly Nd:YAG, KTP, and more recently diode or CO_2 lasers, offers an alternative to conventional scissors or electrosurgery for septum resection. Laser energy allows contact-free, bloodless incision with minimal lateral thermal spread, preserving adjacent endometrium and reducing postoperative adhesions. Modern fiber-delivered diode systems can be introduced through 5-Fr or mini-hysteroscopes, making them suitable for office metroplasty in thin or moderate septa. Key advantages include excellent hemostasis, clear visual fields, and precise depth control. Limitations include high equipment cost, limited availability, and a longer learning curve for safe use.

Combined Approaches

Laparoscopic visualization can be used concurrently to guard against perforation when resecting deep/complete septa or when uterine fundal contour is uncertain. Intraoperative real-time ultrasound (2D or 3D) guidance is an increasingly used adjunct to confirm depth of resection and minimize risk. Recent systematic reviews support intra-operative ultrasound as a useful safety and accuracy tool.

Adhesion Prevention

Evidence for routine use of intrauterine devices, estrogen, or anti-adhesion gels is mixed; hyaluronic acid gels have been used to reduce synechiae in some series, but robust outcome data are limited. Consider on a case-by-case basis.

Energy Settings and Technique Tips

When electrosurgery is used, prefer bipolar energy with normal saline distension when available. Keep resections conservative—cut to the level of normal endometrium and preserve fundal myometrium. Continuous fluid balance monitoring and low-flow settings reduce risks.

End Points of Surgery

(i) Resection or incision up to the fundal level in line with both the ostia and not go deeper. (ii) keep a margin of at least 5 mm from the ostia. (iii) visibility of blood vessels or capillaries or appearance of pinpoint bleeding on reducing intrauterine fluid pressure. (iv) change in color from white of fibrotic septa to salmon pink of healthy tissue.

SPECIAL SITUATIONS: COMPLETE SEPTUM AND ROBERT'S UTERUS

A complete uterine septum extends from the fundal endometrium to the internal cervical os, and in some cases through the cervix and vagina, creating a double or pseudo-didelphic cavity within a single external uterine contour. These anomalies may remain asymptomatic until reproductive challenges arise—most commonly primary infertility, recurrent miscarriage, or preterm labor. In contrast, some women present with obstructive dysmenorrhea when the septum causes asymmetric cavities or partial outflow obstruction.

A rarer but clinically significant variant is the Robert's uterus, defined as a complete septate uterus with one blind (non-communicating) hemi-cavity and one normal communicating cavity. The blind cavity, lined with functional endometrium, accumulates menstrual blood, resulting in unilateral hematometra, severe cyclical pain, or secondary endometriosis from retrograde menstruation.

Guidance with ultrasound or laparoscopy is recommended to avoid perforation, especially in blind hemi-cavity anatomy.

Balloon stents or anti-adhesion gels may be considered in extensive resections.

PRECAUTIONS MITIGATING SURGICAL CHALLENGES AND TECHNICAL PEARLS

- *Guided approach:* For complete septa or Robert's uterus, one can combine hysteroscopy with laparoscopic or transabdominal ultrasound guidance to confirm cavity orientation and prevent fundal perforation.
- *Stepwise incision:* Begin at the lower septal margin and progress upward in small increments until both cavities merge into a unified, symmetrical triangular space. Vaginal septum may be divided with monopolar or bipolar electrocautery. The cervical part may be addressed last as dividing it earlier may cause difficulty in maintaining proper distension. Some prefer to instill dilute methylene blue dye or insert a Foley's catheter in one part of the cavity while resection to aid identification of entry to the other side divided by the septum. In occasional situations, a staged procedure may be performed but usually it can be accomplished in a single sitting.
- *Adhesion prevention:* In extensive resections, consider hyaluronic acid gel or balloon stent placement for 7–10 days, though evidence is mixed.
- *Postoperative imaging:* Repeat 3D-TVUS or office hysteroscopy at 6–8 weeks to confirm normalization of cavity shape and patency of both horns.

When performed with these safeguards, hysteroscopic correction of complete septa and Robert's uterus restores normal uterine anatomy with excellent fertility outcomes and low complication rates.

EXCISION VERSUS RESECTION—CURRENT EVIDENCE

- *Resection/incision (metroplasty by resection or incision):* The traditional hysteroscopic approach where the septum is progressively incised or "shaved" until the uterine cavity assumes a normal contour. This is most commonly performed with a hysteroscopic loop (electrosurgical) or cold scissors. As the septal tissue is incised, the remaining edges retract laterally and the cavity opens—in many cases no bulk tissue needs to be removed. This is the technique described in most classic series and practice guides.

- *Excision (complete removal):* the septum is removed en bloc or in contiguous fragments—the tissue is actively excised from its base so that no gross septal tissue remains. Excision allows retrieval of septal tissue for histopathology and may be favored by some surgeons when the septum is thick, fibromuscular, or when a clear specimen is desired for diagnostic/histologic reasons. Case series and technical reports describe using resectoscope loops, scissors with tissue retrieval, or mechanical tissue-removal devices to accomplish excision.

Network meta-analyses and cohort reviews examine different energy modalities (mechanical vs electrosurgical vs laser) but do not definitively show superior reproductive outcomes for one basic tactic over another—the balance of safety (avoidance of myometrial loss/perforation) and completeness of cavity restoration guides technique choice. Shared decision-making and tailoring to septal morphology remain critical.

POSTOPERATIVE CARE AND FOLLOW-UP

- *Immediate:* Observe for bleeding, fluid imbalance and pain. Routine prophylactic antibiotics are not universally recommended; follow local protocols.
- *Hysteroscopic check:* Many units perform a single diagnostic office hysteroscopy or saline-infusion sonography at 6–12 weeks to exclude residual septum or adhesions in symptomatic patients or when fertility is a priority.
- *Timing of conception:* There is no universal rule; many clinicians advise attempting conception after one normal menstrual cycle and adequate healing, but individualized advice (particularly before ART) is recommended. The ASRM guidance encourages shared decision-making about timing.

COMPLICATIONS AND RISK MITIGATION

Complications include uterine perforation, bleeding, fluid overload (hyponatremia), infection and intrauterine adhesions. Risk mitigation strategies include appropriate energy choice (bipolar where possible), ultrasound or laparoscopic guidance for deeper septa, meticulous fluid monitoring, short stepwise resections and limiting electrosurgical thermal spread. Postoperative surveillance for adhesions in symptomatic or fertility-seeking women permits early hysteroscopic adhesiolysis where needed.

CONCLUSION

Hysteroscopic septum resection remains an important procedure in the gynecologist's armamentarium. The contemporary emphasis is on accurate phenotyping, stratified patient selection, shared decision-making, and using minimally invasive office techniques or image-guided operative approaches where appropriate. Evidence supports benefit in selected patient groups but is not unequivocal for universal resection—practitioners must counsel patients transparently and adopt safety-oriented operative strategies (bipolar energy, intraoperative imaging, fluid monitoring) that reflect recent innovations and guideline recommendations. Continued prospective, well-designed studies will refine which patients derive the greatest reproductive benefit and how best to deliver that care.

SUGGESTED READING

1. Bettocchi S, Nappi L, Ceci O, Selvaggi L. Office hysteroscopy. Obstet Gynecol Clin North Am. 2004;31(3):641-xi.
2. Calabrese S, DE Alberti D, Garuti G. The use of bipolar technology in hysteroscopy. Minerva Ginecol. 2016;68(2):133-42.
3. Carrera M, Pérez Millan F, Alcázar JL, Alonso L, Caballero M, Carugno J, et al. Effect of Hysteroscopic Metroplasty on Reproductive Outcomes in Women with Septate Uterus: Systematic Review and Meta-Analysis. J Minim Invasive Gynecol. 2022;29(4):465-75.
4. Chan YY, Jayaprakasan K, Tan A, Thornton JG, Coomarasamy A, Raine-Fenning NJ. Reproductive outcomes in women with congenital uterine anomalies: a systematic review. Ultrasound Obstet Gynecol. 2011;38(4):371-82.
5. Choe JK, Baggish MS. Hysteroscopic treatment of septate uterus with Neodymium-YAG laser. Fertil Steril. 1992;57(1):81-4.
6. Daniilidis A, Kalpatsanidis A, Kalkan U, Kasmas S, Pados G, Angioni S. Reproductive outcome after operative hysteroscopy for uterine septum: Scissors or diathermy?. Minerva Ginecol. 2020;72(1):36-42.
7. Di Spiezio Sardo A, Di Carlo C, Minozzi S, Spinelli M, Pistotti V, Alviggi C, et al. Efficacy of hysteroscopy in improving reproductive outcomes of infertile couples: a systematic review and meta-analysis. Hum Reprod Update. 2016;22(4):479-96.
8. Etrusco A, Buzzaccarini G, Laganà AS, Chiantera V, Vitale SG, Angioni S, et al. Use of Diode Laser in Hysteroscopy for the Management of Intrauterine Pathology: A Systematic Review. Diagnostics (Basel). 2024;14(3):327.
9. Fei Z, Bin Z, Xin X, Fei H, Yuechong C. Meta-analysis on the use of hyaluronic acid gel to prevent recurrence of intrauterine adhesion after hysteroscopic adhesiolysis. Taiwan J Obstet Gynecol. 2019;58(6):731-6.
10. Grimbizis GF, Gordts S, Di Spiezio Sardo A, Brucker S, De Angelis C, Gergolet M, et al. The ESHRE/ESGE consensus on the classification of female genital tract congenital anomalies. Hum Reprod. 2013;28(8):2032-44.
11. Homer HA, Li TC, Cooke ID. The septate uterus: a review of management and reproductive outcome. Fertil Steril. 2000;73(1):1-14.
12. Jansen FW, Vredevoogd CB, van Ulzen K, Hermans J, Trimbos JB, Trimbos-Kemper TC. Complications of hysteroscopy: a prospective, multicenter study. Obstet Gynecol. 2000;96(2):266-70.

13. Jiang Y, Wang L, Wang B, Shen H, Wu J, He J, et al. Reproductive outcomes of natural pregnancy after hysteroscopic septum resection in patients with a septate uterus: a systematic review and meta-analysis. Am J Obstet Gynecol MFM. 2023;5(1):100762.
14. Litta P, Leggieri C, Conte L, Dalla Toffola A, Multinu F, Angioni S. Monopolar versus bipolar device: safety, feasibility, limits and perioperative complications in performing hysteroscopic myomectomy. Clin Exp Obstet Gynecol. 2014;41(3):335-8.
15. Litta P, Pozzan C, Merlin F, Sacco G, Saccardi C, Ambrosini G, et al. Hysteroscopic Metroplasty under Laparoscopic Guidance in Infertile Women with Septate Uteri: Follow-up of Reproductive Outcome. J Reprod Med. 2004;49(4):274-8.
16. Ludwin A, Martins WP, Nastri CO, Ludwin I, Coelho Neto MA, Leitão VM, et al. Congenital Uterine Malformation by Experts (CUME): better criteria for distinguishing between normal/arcuate and septate uterus? Ultrasound Obstet Gynecol. 2018;51(1):101-9.
17. Ludwin A, Pityński K, Ludwin I, Banas T, Knafel A. Two- and three-dimensional ultrasonography and sonohysterography versus hysteroscopy with laparoscopy in the differential diagnosis of septate, bicornuate, and arcuate uteri. J Minim Invasive Gynecol. 2013;20(1):90-9.
18. Practice Committee of the American Society for Reproductive Medicine. Electronic address: ASRM@asrm.org; Practice Committee of the American Society for Reproductive Medicine. Uterine septum: a guideline. Fertil Steril. 2016;106(3):530-40.
19. Practice Committee of the American Society for Reproductive Medicine. Electronic address: asrm@asrm.org. Evidence-based diagnosis and treatment for uterine septum: a guideline. Fertil Steril. 2024;122(2):251-65.
20. Rikken JFW, Kowalik CR, Emanuel MH, Bongers MY, Spinder T, Jansen FW, et al. Septum resection versus expectant management in women with a septate uterus: an international multicentre open-label randomized controlled trial. Hum Reprod. 2021;36(5):1260-7.
21. Salim R, Woelfer B, Backos M, Regan L, Jurkovic D. Reproducibility of three-dimensional ultrasound diagnosis of congenital uterine anomalies. Ultrasound Obstet Gynecol. 2003;21(6):578-82.
22. Troiano RN, McCarthy SM. Mullerian duct anomalies: imaging and clinical issues. Radiology. 2004;233(1):19-34.
23. Valle RF, Ekpo GE. Hysteroscopic metroplasty for the septate uterus: review and meta-analysis. J Minim Invasive Gynecol. 2013;20(1):22-42.
24. Valle RF. Hysteroscopic treatment of partial and complete uterine septum. Int J Fertil Menopausal Stud. 1996;41(3):310-5.
25. Venetis CA, Papadopoulos SP, Campo R, Gordts S, Tarlatzis BC, Grimbizis GF. Clinical implications of congenital uterine anomalies: a meta-analysis of comparative studies. Reprod Biomed Online. 2014;29(6):665-83.

20 CHAPTER

Hysteroscopic Removal of Intrauterine Foreign Bodies: Principles and Practice

Kalpana Choudhury

Hysteroscopy has revolutionized intrauterine diagnosis and therapy, providing a safe and precise alternative to blind surgical procedures. Among its many indications, the removal of intrauterine foreign bodies—ranging from retained intrauterine devices (IUDs) to bone fragments or surgical material—represents an important clinical skill. Endoscopic surgeons should be equipped with evidence-based knowledge to perform safe, effective, and fertility-preserving hysteroscopic foreign body removal.

INTRODUCTION

Intrauterine foreign bodies (IUFBs) may arise from misplaced contraceptive devices, retained fetal bones, surgical gauze, suture material, or migration of devices from surrounding structures etc. These can lead to abnormal uterine bleeding, infertility, chronic pelvic pain, or recurrent infection. Hysteroscopy provides direct visualization of the uterine cavity, allowing precise localization and complete removal of such foreign materials with minimal trauma and reduced complications **(Tables 1 and 2)**.

INDICATIONS FOR HYSTEROSCOPIC REMOVAL

- Retained fetal bones **(Fig. 1)**, Product of conception **(Fig. 2)**, following abortion or miscarriage

TABLE 1: Preoperative evaluation.

Parameter	*Investigation/assessment*	*Purpose*
Clinical history	Menstrual irregularities, infertility, pelvic pain	Identify symptoms and possible cause
Ultrasonography	Transvaginal or 3D imaging	Localization of foreign body
Hysterosalpingography (HSG)	When ultrasound is inconclusive	Detect cavity distortion
Laboratory tests	CBC, RBS, TSH, infection screening	Preoperative fitness
Informed consent	Explanation of risks and outcomes	Medico-legal and ethical compliance

TABLE 2: Types of intrauterine foreign bodies and hysteroscopic management.

Type of foreign body	*Common cause*	*Hysteroscopic approach*
Retained IUD or fragment	Breakage during removal	Grasping forceps under direct vision
Fetal bone fragments	Missed postabortion tissue	Loop resection or forceps extraction
Suture material	Previous uterine surgery	Cut and remove under vision
Gauze or sponge	Retained surgical item	Grasp and extract carefully
Tubal stent or device	Migration	Identify, dislodge, remove gently

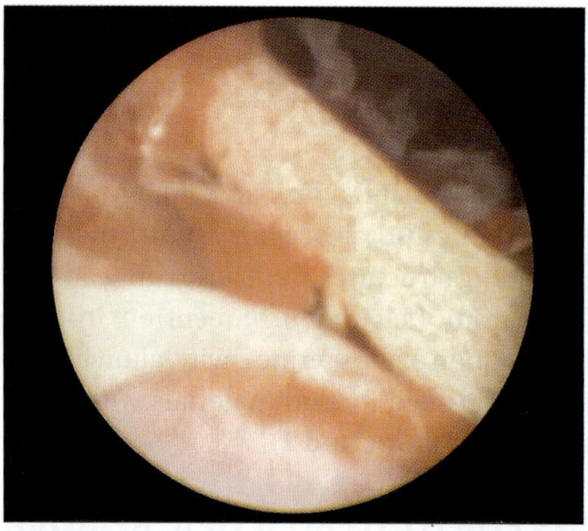

Fig. 1: Retained fetal bone.

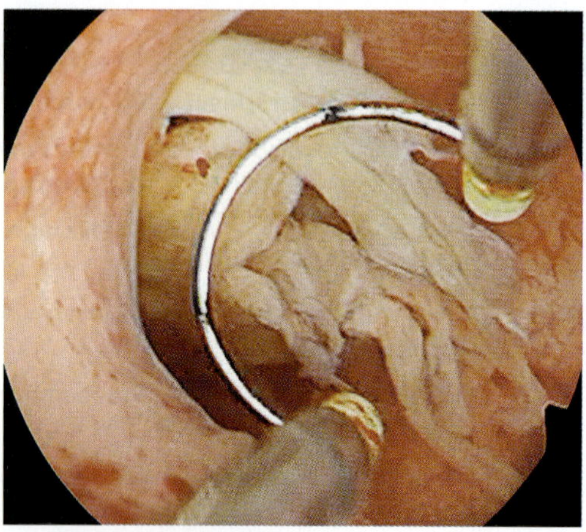

Fig. 2: Retained product of conception.

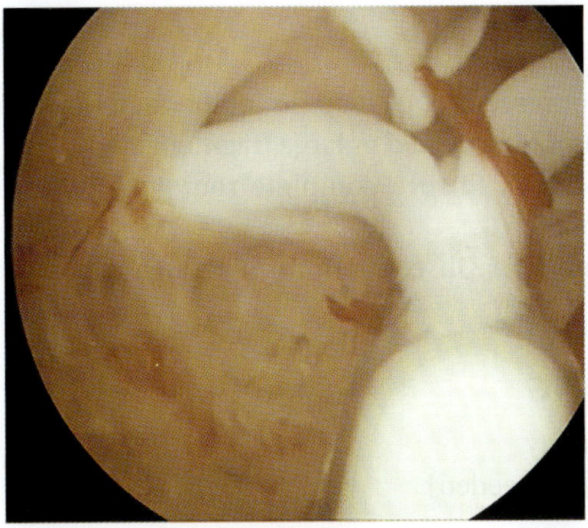

Fig. 3: Retained Cu T.

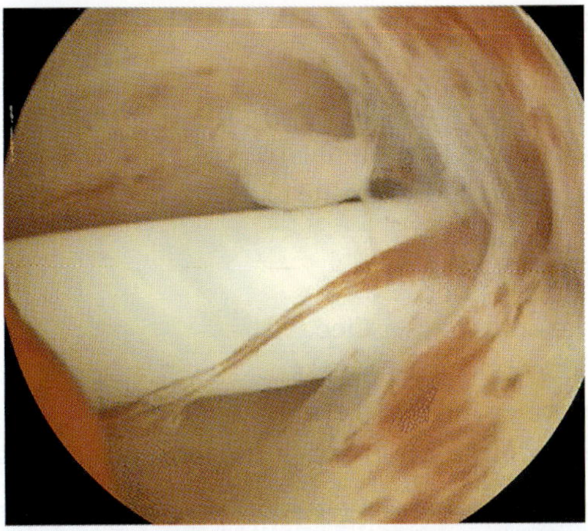

Fig. 4: Retained Cu T.

- Retained or fragmented intrauterine contraceptive devices (IUDs) **(Figs. 3 and 4)**
- Foreign bodies after uterine surgery (e.g., sutures, gauze)
- Calcified endometrial deposits or migrated tubal stents
- Post surgical materials following myomectomy or cesarean section.

HYSTEROSCOPIC TECHNIQUE

- *Anesthesia:* Usually performed under paracervical block or short general anesthesia.
- *Cervical preparation:* Gradual dilation with Hegar's dilators or use of misoprostol for softening.
- *Distension medium:* Normal saline (preferred for bipolar system).
- *Hysteroscopic visualization:* Introduction of diagnostic or operative hysteroscope to identify the foreign body.

- *Removal Instruments:*
  - Grasping forceps
  - Scissors or resectoscope loop (for embedded fragments)
  - Morcellator for calcified or large fragments
- *Cavity inspection:* Ensure complete removal and intact endometrial lining.
- *Postprocedure care:* Observation for bleeding or infection; antibiotics if indicated.

MONITORING

- Ultrasonography
- Laparoscopy (If needed)

COMPLICATIONS

- Uterine perforation
- Bleeding or infection
- Incomplete removal leading to persistence of symptoms
- Fluid overload (if using hypotonic distension media)
- Rarely, Asherman's syndrome due to aggressive curettage

POSTOPERATIVE CARE

- Analgesics and antibiotics as needed
- Follow-up ultrasound at 2–4 weeks
- Hysteroscopic re-evaluation if symptoms persist
- Counseling on contraception and future fertility planning

KEY POINTS

- Direct visualization via hysteroscopy ensures complete and safe removal of intrauterine foreign bodies.
- Use of normal saline with bipolar instruments minimizes fluid-related complications.
- Preoperative imaging helps localize the foreign body and plan the approach.
- Postoperative follow-up is essential to prevent recurrence or intrauterine adhesions.

SUGGESTED READING

1. Baggish MS, Valle RF. Atlas of Hysteroscopy, 5th edition. London: CRC Press; 2020.
2. Bettocchi S, Nappi L, Ceci O, Selvaggi L. Hysteroscopic management of foreign bodies in the uterine cavity. J Am Assoc Gynecol Laparosc. 2004;11(2):207-11.
3. Gimpelson RJ. Hysteroscopic foreign body retrieval: A minimally invasive approach. Obstet Gynecol Clin North Am. 2021;48(4):797-809.
4. Jayakrishnan K, Al-Salhi S. Retained intrauterine fetal bone fragments: An unusual cause of secondary infertility. J Obstet Gynaecol Res. 2015;41(6):988-92.
5. Valle RF, Sciarra JJ. Hysteroscopic removal of intrauterine foreign bodies. Fertil Steril. 1980;34(3):258-61.

CHAPTER 21

Diagnosis of Female Genital Tuberculosis/Koch's by Hysteroscopy

Priya Bhave Chittawar, Mrinal Chatterjee

INTRODUCTION AND DEFINITION

Female genital tuberculosis (FGTB) is a chronic granulomatous infection caused by *Mycobacterium tuberculosis*, affecting primarily women of reproductive age. It remains an important but often underdiagnosed cause of infertility in India, contributing to 5–19% of infertility cases depending on region and population risk profiles.

Due to its paucibacillary nature, the disease often presents silently, leading to delayed diagnosis and substantial reproductive morbidity. Most cases arise from hematogenous spread of pulmonary or extragenital tuberculosis. FGTB predominantly affects:

- *Fallopian tubes:* 90–100%
- *Endometrium:* 50–60%
- *Ovaries:* 20–30%
- *Cervix:* 5–15%
- *Vagina/vulva:* Rare

Recent literature highlights that FGTB is a modifiable burden in fertility practice, and diagnosis requires a multimodal approach—combining hysteroscopy, laparoscopy, molecular assays (GeneXpert, PCR), microbiology, and histopathology.

Hysteroscopy offers direct visualization of characteristic endometrial alterations and enables targeted biopsy, significantly enhancing diagnostic accuracy, particularly in early or atypical cases. Prompt diagnosis and timely antitubercular therapy (ATT) may limit irreversible damage and preserve reproductive potential.

EPIDEMIOLOGY

FGTB is prevalent in South Asia, including India, Pakistan, Nepal, Afghanistan, and parts of Africa. It is most common in women aged 20–40 years, coinciding with peak fertility.

Risk Factors

- Prior pulmonary or extrapulmonary TB
- Family history of TB
- Low socioeconomic status, malnutrition

- Close household TB contact
- Immunosuppression
- Previous pelvic infections
- Residence in TB-endemic areas
  FGTB contributes to 19–40% of infertility in high-burden regions.

PATHOPHYSIOLOGY AND SITES INVOLVED

The infection spreads hematogenously, occasionally lymphatically or through direct extension.

Tubal involvement causes:
- Tubal blockage
- Beading, rigid tubes
- Hydrosalpinx
- Tubo-ovarian masses

Endometrial involvement leads to:
- Thin, pale endometrium
- Adhesions
- Asherman-like cavity
- Poor vascularity → impaired implantation

CLINICAL PRESENTATION

FGTB may be asymptomatic or mimic chronic pelvic pathology.

When to suspect FGTB?

Reproductive Symptoms:
- Primary/secondary infertility (most common)
- Thin endometrium (<6 mm) unresponsive to therapy
- Recurrent implantation failure (RIF)
- Recurrent pregnancy loss (RPL)

Menstrual Dysfunction:
- Hypomenorrhea
- Oligomenorrhoea
- Amenorrhea
- Post-menstrual spotting

Chronic Pelvic Symptoms:
- Chronic pelvic pain
- Dysmenorrhea
- Chronic endometritis-like symptoms

Radiological Clues ***(Figs. 1 and 2):***
- Calcified tubes
- Distorted cavity
- Hydrosalpinx

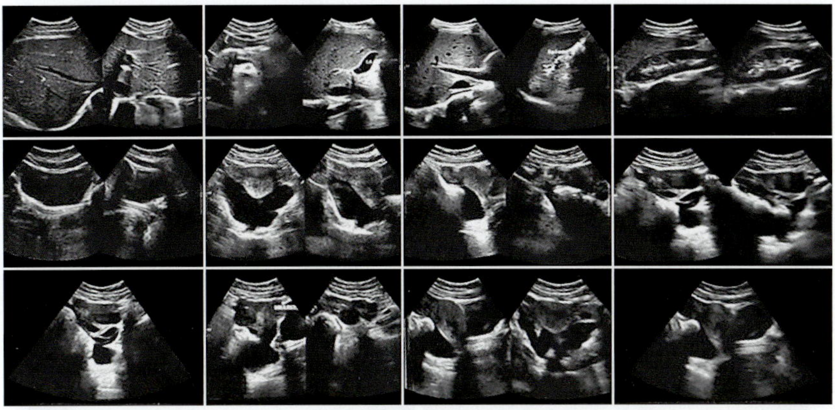

Fig. 1: *USG (Abdomen + Pelvis)* s/o Normal sized uterus with 6.3 mm thin endometrium, right ovary—bulky. Left ovary—unilocular cyst—42 × 39 × 29 mm size cyst lumen, few soft echoes. App. 147cc of collection in the pelvis in both the adnexa and cul de sac. Few thin septations in the collection forming inclusion cyst. A pocket of collection in left adnexa anteriorly is full ground glass echoes. App. 52cc.

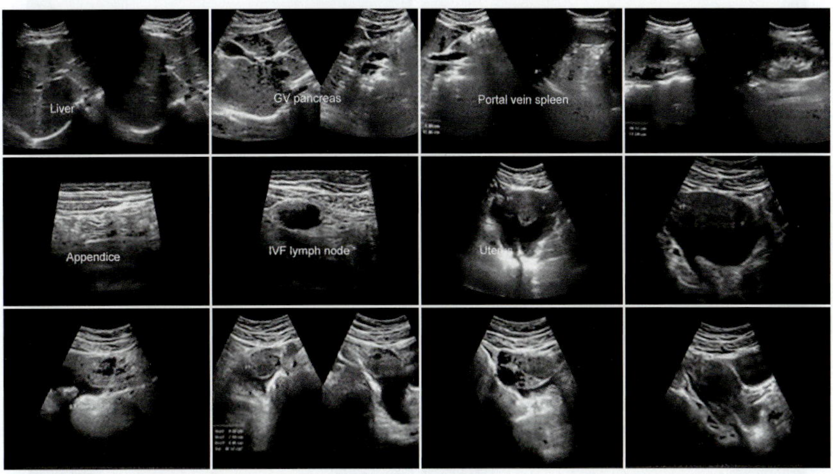

Fig. 2: *USG (Abdomen + Pelvis):* Grossly normal Upper abdomen, Both ovaries adhered to body of uterus with antero-medal fixity. Complex solid-cystic tubo-ovarian masses in both adnexa with cystic component revealing low level echos. The Adnexal lesions are surrounded by walled off fluid collections of 30–40cc on each side. Mild diffuse omental thickening seen in pelvic cavity with small hypoechoic omental nodules one anteriorly and one in RIF. A hypoechoic nodule with speckled calcification seen in POD. Plan to continue AKT for 3 more months.

DIAGNOSTIC APPROACH

Because no single test is diagnostic, a composite approach is essential.

Baseline Imaging:

- *HSG:* Beading, rigid "pipe-stem" tubes

- *USG:* Hydrosalpinx, adnexal masses
- *MRI:* Useful for differential diagnosis

ROLE OF HYSTEROSCOPY IN DIAGNOSIS OF FGTB

Hysteroscopy is critical because it allows direct visualization of subtle endometrial pathology and enables targeted biopsies.

What hysteroscopy assesses (Figs. 3A to F)?

- Endometrial texture, vascularity, and thickness
- Synechiae/Asherman's syndrome

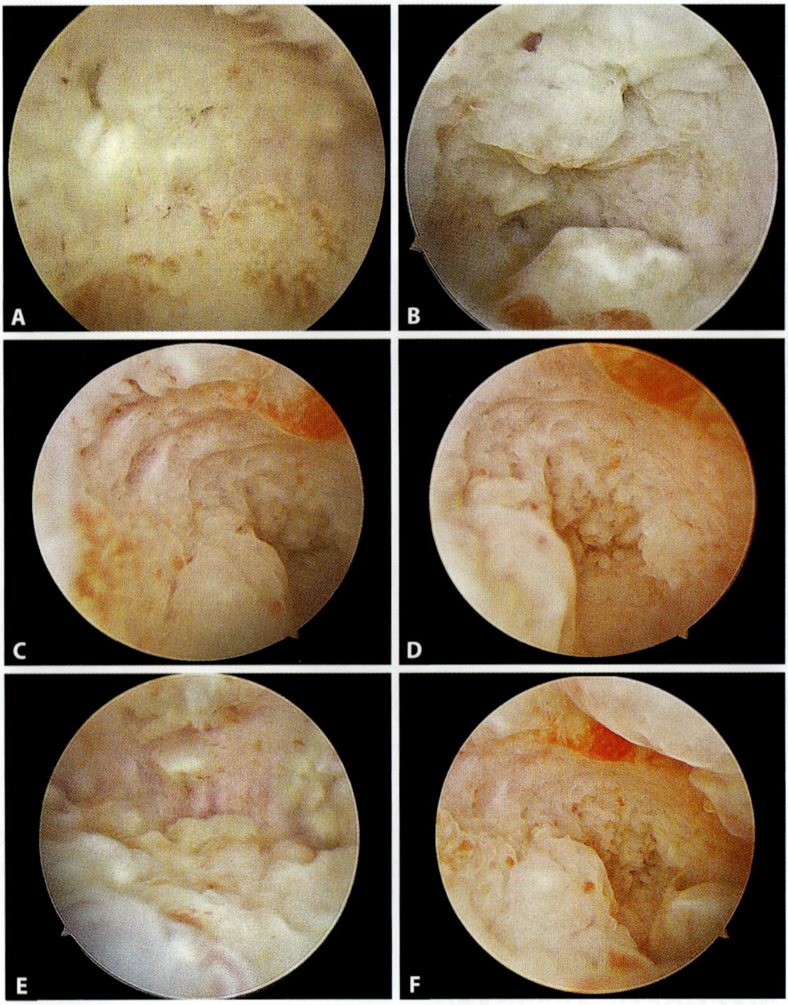

Figs. 3A to F: Intraoperative Hysteroscopic Pictures A-F s/o Tubercular endometritis. (A) Right Ostia with periosteal fibrosis; (B) Left Ostia periosteal fibrosis, caseation; (C) Pale Endometrium with poor vascularity; (D) Yellow Necrotic patches; (E) Caseation; and (F) Micro polyps.

- Tubal ostial morphology
- Presence of granulomas or caseous foci
- Cavity distortion
- Stenosis of cervical canal

Targeted biopsies from pale areas, granulomas, and adhesions significantly improve detection, outperforming blind biopsies.

Endoscopic findings form a major component of diagnostic bundles recommended in recent guidelines.

Hysteroscopic Findings Suggestive of Genital TB

(Refer to **Table 1** for Findings during Hysteroscopy and their Description).

(Refer to **Table 2** for Evidence Based Studies).

Endometrial Findings

- Pale, avascular endometrium
- Reduced vascularity; poor bleeding points
- Cobweb pattern (patchy fibrosis)
- Caseous deposits (yellow-white plaques)
- Whitish granulomas
- Rough, necrotic patches
- Poor cavity distensibility

Adhesions/Synechiae

- Filmy or dense adhesions
- Central cavity obliteration (late stage)
- T-shaped or small cavity from fibrosis

Tubal Ostial Changes

- Pinpoint, slit-like, or obliterated ostia
- Beaded outline
- "Tobacco-pouch" appearance

TABLE 1: Hysteroscopic features of FGTB **(Figs. 3A to F)**.

Finding	*Description*
Pale endometrium	Thin, avascular, patchy pallor
Caseous necrosis	Yellowish-white cheesy areas
Granulomas	Small raised white nodules
Synechiae	Filmy/dense adhesions; cavity distortion
Tubal ostia changes	Pinpoint, beaded, or obliterated ostia
Cervical stenosis	Narrow/fibrotic canal

TABLE 2: Evidence summary.

Study	*Design/Sample*	*Key Diagnostic Findings*	*Clinical Implications*
Mondal et al., 2023	Large case series; 16,784 infertile women; 309 confirmed FGTB	Pale endometrium, dense IU adhesions, hydrosalpinx, tubercles, tubo-ovarian masses	Hystero-laparoscopy provides strong diagnostic clues; essential before ART
Sharma et al., 2023	Diagnostic accuracy study in infertile women	PCR more sensitive than culture; GeneXpert highly specific but low sensitivity	Molecular tests must be paired with biopsy; GeneXpert negative ≠ rule out FGTB
Indian Pelvic TB Review, 2022	Review of Indian cohorts	Laparoscopy detects early pelvic TB missed on imaging; hysteroscopy shows fibrosis and caseous lesions	Laparoscopy acts as practical gold standard for pelvic TB in endemic regions
Hysteroscopy Review (BJOG)	Overview of hysteroscopic findings	Pale cavity, starry-sky tubercles, distorted cavity, fibrosis	Hysteroscopy is critical for assessing cavity and predicting ART outcomes
Tubal TB Cohort Data (PGIMER/AIIMS/NIMS)	Tubal factor infertility groups	TB associated with hydrosalpinx, fimbrial block, frozen pelvis	ATT + salpingectomy improves IVF success; tubal damage often permanent

- Flame-shaped ostia
- Surrounding mucosal scarring

Cervical Findings

- Cervical stenosis
- Fibrotic internal os

Rare Findings

- Endometrial calcifications
- Pockets of pus/microabscesses
- Pyometra

**Findings validated by BJOG Case Series (2023; $n = 16,784$) **

- Pale endometrium
- Mucosal whitening
- Micro polyps
- Tubercles/caseous foci
- Adhesions
- Distorted cavity

  These were significantly associated with confirmed FGTB.

MICROBIOLOGICAL AND HISTOLOGICAL TESTING

Target Biopsy Sites **(Figs. 3A to F)**:

- Pale/whitish areas
- Granulomas
- Adhesions
- Caseous/necrotic patches

Recommended Tests:

Microbiology

- CBNAAT/GeneXpert MTB/RIF → rapid, specific
- TB PCR → high sensitivity
- MGIT culture → gold standard (low positivity in paucibacillary disease)
- AFB smear

Histopathology

- Epithelioid granulomas
- Langhans giant cells
- Caseous necrosis

Evidence: Hysteroscopy-guided biopsy improves diagnostic yield (PMID: 37973605).

DIFFERENTIAL DIAGNOSIS

- Chronic endometritis
- IU adhesions from curettage
- Asherman syndrome
- Post-PID scarring
- Endometrial atrophy
- Uterine anomalies
- Submucous fibroids/polyps

DIAGNOSTIC ALGORITHM (CLINICAL + ENDOSCOPY + LAB)

- High clinical suspicion→ USG/HSG
- Diagnostic hysteroscopy **(Figs. 3A to F, Table 2)**
  - If pale mucosa/adhesions/granulomas → targeted biopsy
- Send specimens for:
  - HPE
  - GeneXpert/PCR
  - AFB smear
  - MGIT culture
- Diagnosis confirmed if:
  - HPE showing granulomas OR

  - GeneXpert/PCR positive OR
  - Culture positive
  - Classical finding on hysteroscopy
- Start ATT as per NTEP guidelines
- Reassess fertility at 6–9 months

Let's see a case for an example. A 22 years old unmarried female presented with on and off mild abdominal pain. USG **(Fig. 1)** and MRI done with features suggestive of chronic inflammatory/ infective etiology with B/L TO masses. Proceeded with Diagnostic Hysterolaparoscopy **(Figs. 3A to F)** with findings confirmed. Blood, HPE, Microbiological Tests all were negative. Started on ATT. After 6 months of ATT Patient had relief of symptoms, Post 6 months USG **(Fig. 2)** was done and was continued ATT for 3 more months.

COMPOSITE CRITERIA FOR DIAGNOSIS

Major

- CBNAAT/Culture positive
- HPE granulomas
- Classic hysteroscopic findings
- Laparoscopic evidence

Minor

- PCR positive
- Imaging suggestive
- Menstrual abnormalities
- Thin endometrium
- Past TB history

Diagnosis: ≥1 Major OR ≥2 Minor + strong clinical suspicion

MANAGEMENT OF FGTB

Medical Treatment

- ATT Category I regimen (2HRZE + 4HRE) for 6 months
- Add supportive therapy
  - High-protein diet
  - NSAIDs
  - Hematinics

Surgical Treatment

Indications

- Hydrosalpinx before IVF
- Persistent tubo-ovarian mass

- Severe adhesions
- Complications (e.g., pyometra)

Infertility Management

- Natural conception possible only in early disease
- Permanent tubal damage → IVF/ICSI required
- Remove/occlude hydrosalpinx before IVF
- Severe endometrial scarring → poor prognosis

Endometrial rehabilitation

- Hysteroscopic adhesiolysis
- PRP/G-CSF (limited evidence)

PROGNOSIS

- *Tubal disease:* largely irreversible
- Endometrial involvement determines fertility outcomes
- Implantation failure common even after ATT
- Severe fibrosis → guarded prognosis

CONCLUSION

FGTB is a preventable and modifiable cause of infertility in India.

Hysteroscopy plays a central role in diagnosis, offering real-time visualization of hallmark features and enabling high-yield targeted biopsies. A multimodal diagnostic approach combining endoscopy, molecular assays, microbiology, and histopathology provides the best accuracy. Early diagnosis and timely ATT can mitigate long-term reproductive impairment, although advanced cases may continue to have poor fertility outcomes.

KEY POINTS

- FGTB requires a high index of suspicion in infertility.
- Hysteroscopy demonstrates characteristic features: pale endometrium, adhesions, caseous deposits, granulomas, tubal ostial abnormalities.
- Targeted hysteroscopic biopsy + GeneXpert/PCR/HPE = highest diagnostic accuracy.
- Early detection is essential to prevent irreversible reproductive damage.

SUGGESTED READING

1. Baloch S, et al. Role of hysteroscopy in diagnosis of endometrial TB. Int J Reprod Contracept Obstet Gynecol. 2017.
2. Endometrial damage outcomes in FGTB. Fertil Steril. 2014.
3. Garg P, Mehta R, Sharma R, et al. Female genital tuberculosis in subfertile women: a large case series. BJOG. 2023.

4. Grace GA, et al. Modern diagnosis of genital tuberculosis. J Clin Tuberc Other Mycobact Dis. 2017.
5. Hysteroscopy Review. BJOG Online Library. 2023.
6. Indian Pelvic TB Review. ResearchGate publication ID 397741. 2022.
7. Kriplani A, et al. Endometrial tuberculosis and infertility. Fertil Steril. 2014.
8. Mondal R, Jaiswal N, Bhave Chittawar P, Mandal P. Laparoscopic and hysteroscopic findings in women with subfertility and tuberculosis. BJOG. 2024;131(7):929-40.
9. Mondal R, Nandi M, Iqbal I, Bhave Chittawar P. Breaking the Silence on Female Genital Tuberculosis: A Modifiable Burden in Fertility Care. J Obstet Gynaecol Res. 2025;51(11):e70131.
10. Sharma JB, et al. Genital tuberculosis in women. Indian J Med Res. 2018.
11. Sharma JB, Singh N, et al. Diagnostic performance of PCR and GeneXpert in endometrial tuberculosis among infertile women. Int J Gynaecol Obstet. 2023.
12. Sultan AE, et al. Female genital tuberculosis among infertile women: meta-analysis. Sultan Qaboos Univ Med J. 2022.
13. Tripathy SN, et al. Hysteroscopic findings in female genital tuberculosis. J Obstet Gynaecol India. 2012.
14. Tubal TB Cohort Data from PGIMER/AIIMS/NIMS (2018–2022).

CHAPTER 22

Office Hysteroscopy

Tanvir Singh, R Hepshiba

INTRODUCTION

Office hysteroscopy is a minimally invasive, diagnostic and therapeutic procedure that allows direct visualization of the endometrial cavity without the need for general anesthesia or operating theatre infrastructure. It has revolutionized outpatient gynecology by enhancing diagnostic accuracy and offering real-time treatment options with minimal discomfort and high patient satisfaction.

PATIENT PREPARATION

- *Informed consent:* Clearly explain procedure, benefits, risks, and alternatives.
- *Timing:* Optimal during proliferative phase (Day 6–10 of cycle).
- *Premedication:* NSAIDs (e.g., ibuprofen 400 mg) 30–60 minutes prior to reduce discomfort.
- *Bladder:* Should be partially filled for ease of scope entry.

PROCEDURE

Basic steps of office hysteroscopy **(Figs. 1 to 4; Flowchart 1)**.

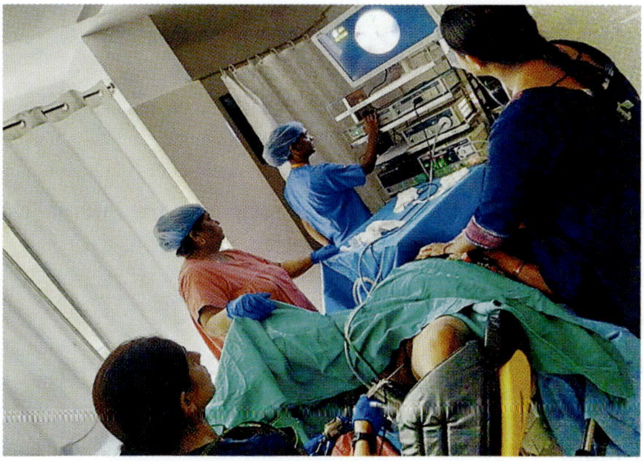

Fig. 1: Patient preparation and position.

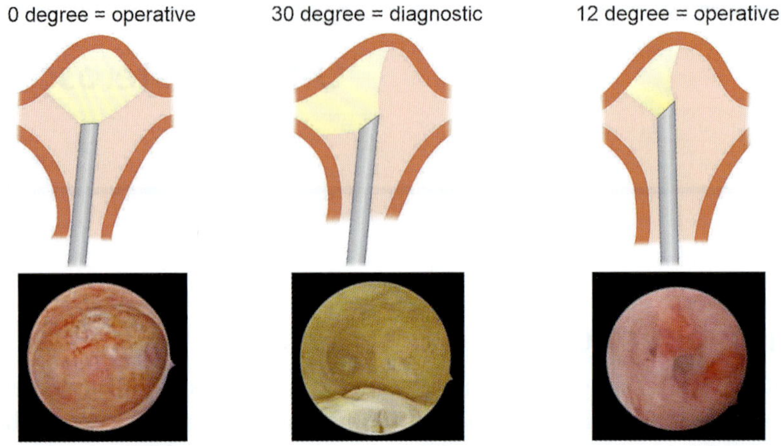

Fig. 2: Types of hysteroscopic camera: 0 degree: Primarily used for operative hysteroscopy, offering a direct end-on view. 30 degree: Ideal for diagnostic purposes, providing a broader visual field. 12 degree: An alternative for operative procedures with moderate angular visualization.
Source: Wright KN, Curr Obstet Gynecol Rep (2024).

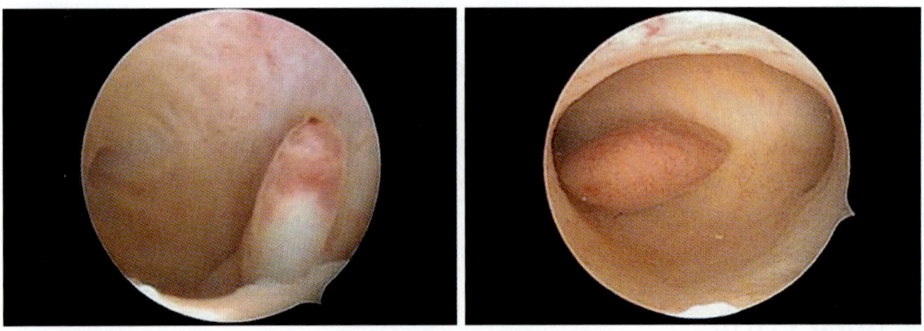

Fig. 3: Camera orientation. Stable hand control and camera alignment improve procedural efficiency and image quality.

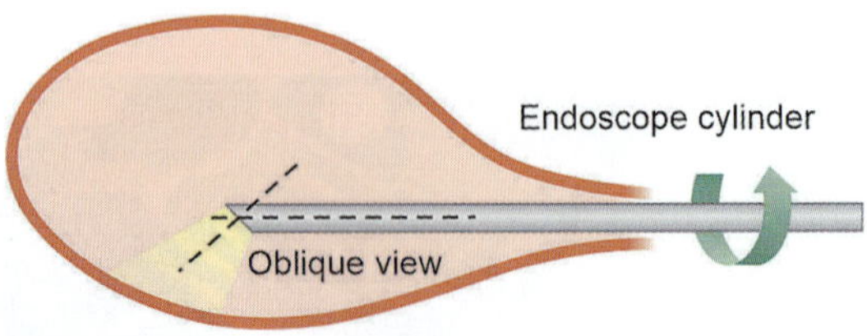

Fig. 4: For oblique view. Position the scope to align with the internal os and maintain an oval profile for better navigation.

PAIN MANAGEMENT AND TOLERANCE

Pain is the primary barrier to successful office hysteroscopy.

Factors influencing discomfort:
- Scope diameter
- Vaginoscopic vs. speculum technique

Flowchart 1: Basic steps of office hysteroscopy.

Step 1: Patient positioning
Lithotomy position with privacy and support. Drape appropriately

↓

Step 2: Vaginoscopic approach
Preferred over traditional speculum method to reduce pain. Insert hysteroscope directly into the vagina, advance through cervix under vision

↓

Step 3: Uterine cavity inspection
Examine systematically:
• Cervical canal • Uterine fundus • Lateral walls • Ostia • Endometrial surface

↓

Step 4: Targeted intervention (If Indicated)
Polyps, adhesions, or septa can be addressed using operative tools via the working channel

↓

Step 5: Documentation and counseling
Capture images/videos. Provide patient explanation, results, and follow-up plan

- Uterine orientation
- Parity

Use of small-diameter hysteroscopes, slow insufflation, and minimizing cervical manipulation improves tolerance.

Analgesia

- Most cases require none; Level 1–3a analgesia may be used (NSAIDs ± paracervical block)
- *Pain tolerates tool:*
- *VAS (Visual analogue scale of pain):* 0-10 scale of subjective pain

Diagnostic Accuracy and Advantages

- Superior to blind procedures (e.g., D&C)
- Real-time visualization
- Ability to biopsy or treat in same sitting
- Minimal downtime
- No general anesthesia required

Sensitivity and specificity for intrauterine pathologies exceed 90% in expert hands.

Table 1 *gives the indications of office hysteroscopy.*

Table 2 *gives the information regarding equipment and setup.*

Timely hysteroscopy improves clinical decision-making and reduces unnecessary interventions.

Max isotonic fluid deficit: 2,500 mL (750 mL if comorbidities); rare in office.

TABLE 1: Indications.

Diagnostic	*Operative*
Abnormal uterine bleeding (AUB)	Polypectomy
Infertility/recurrent pregnancy loss	Adhesiolysis
Postmenopausal bleeding	Myomectomy (Type 0–I)
Abnormal ultrasound findings	Retained products removal
Foreign body localization	Endometrial sampling under vision
	Congenital uterine anomalies

TABLE 2: Equipment and setup (Figs. 5A to D).

Component	*Specifications/Notes*
Hysteroscope	1.9–2.9 mm continuous-flow (most common)
Optics	0° or 30° lens
Light Source	LED/Xenon
Camera & Monitoring	HD camera with recording capability (preferable)
Distension Medium	Normal saline [for bipolar/hysteroscopic tissue removal system (HTRS)]
Fluid Delivery	Gravity or pump (80–100 mm Hg)
Instruments	Graspers, scissors, bipolar electrodes/mini-resectoscope/HTRS

A

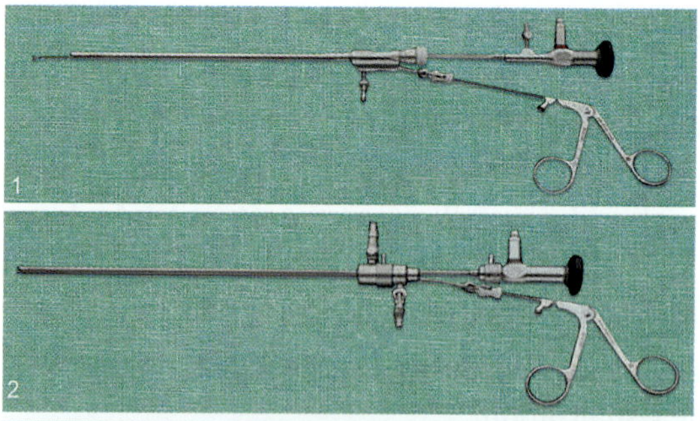

B

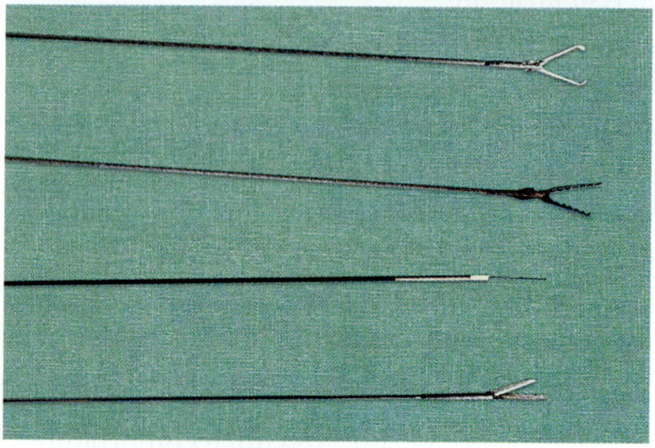

Figs. 5A and B

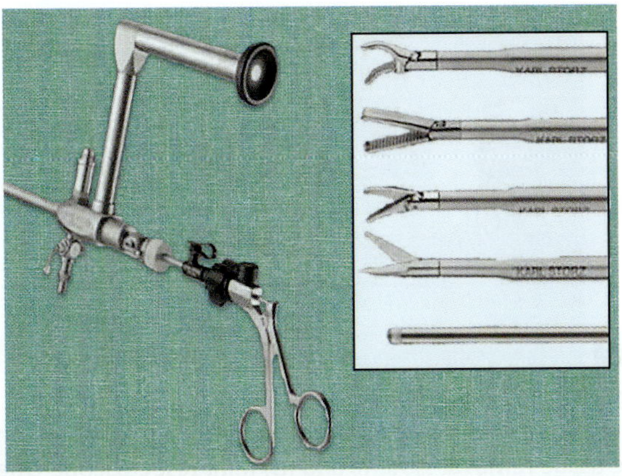

C1

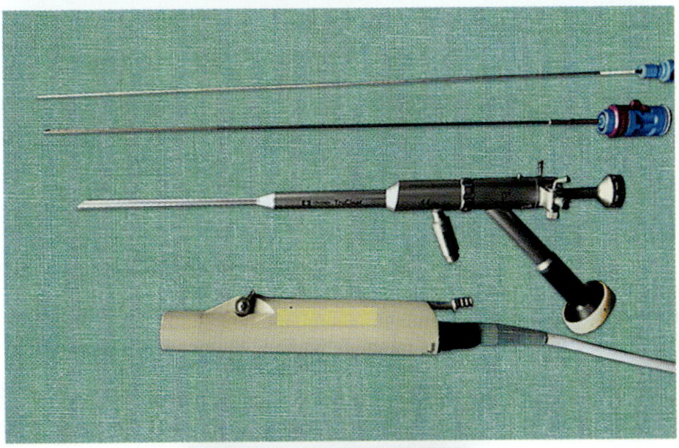

C2

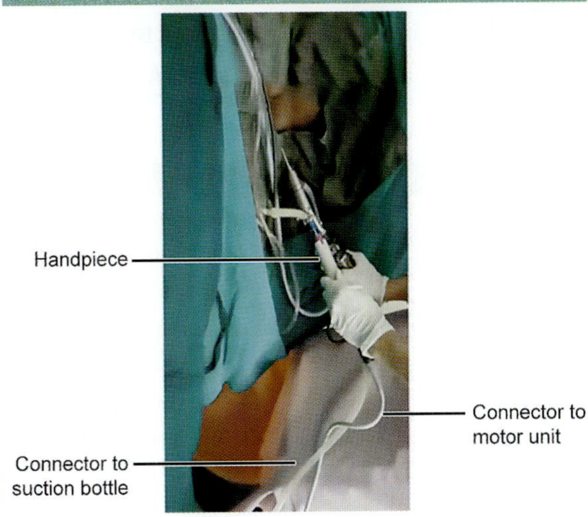

C3

Figs. 5C1 to C3

D
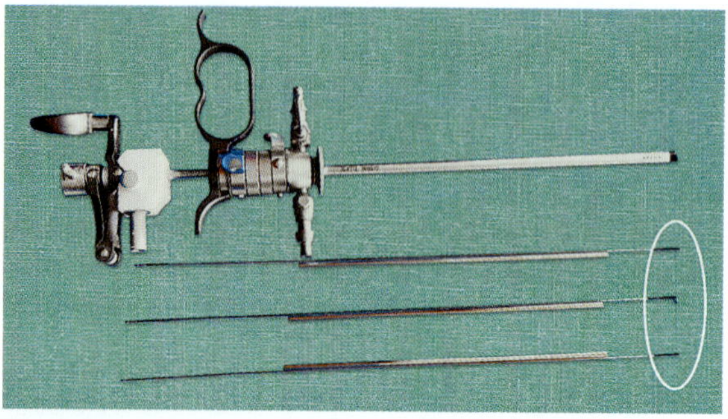

Figs. 5A to D: Instrument—Hysteroscope. (A) Sizes from 1.9 to 2.8 mm; 4 to 5; Rigid/Flexible; (B) 5 Fr instruments semi-rigid Reusable, 35-40 cm length; (C: 1-3) Hysteroscopic tissue removal system; and (D) Mini-resectoscope Operative Procedures in Office Setting.

TABLE 3: Operative Procedures in office setting.

Lesion	*Management*
Endometrial polyp	Polypectomy **(Fig. 6)**
Septum	Resection (if symptomatic) **(Figs. 7A to D)**
Submucosal fibroid	Enucleation/morcellation/Resection (if feasible) **(Figs. 8A to D)**
Retained products of conception	Mechanical/ morcellation/ resection **(Figs. 9A to F)**
Endometrial hyperplasia	Biopsy **(Figs. 10A and B)**
Adhesions (Asherman's)	Adhesiolysis **(Figs. 11A to D)**

TABLE 4: Complications and prevention.

Complications	*Prevention*
Pain/VVS	Counseling, vaginoscopy entry
Perforation	Gentle technique
Bleeding	Low pressure, bipolar energy
Infection	Aseptic technique
Fluid overload	Monitor inflow-outflow balance

Summary: Office hysteroscopy is a safe, effective, and patient-centered diagnostic and therapeutic procedure that can be performed without anesthesia by trained clinicians.

***Table 3** will tell us about the operative procedure for the given diagnosis in office setting.*

***Table 4** will explain about the complications during procedure and how to tackle/prevent such complication.*

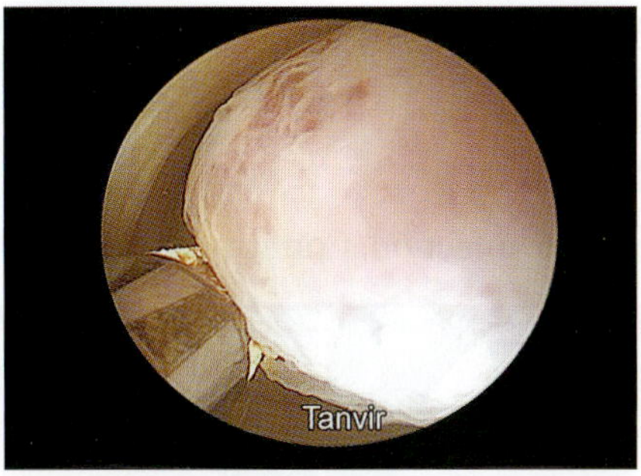

Fig. 6: Polyps.

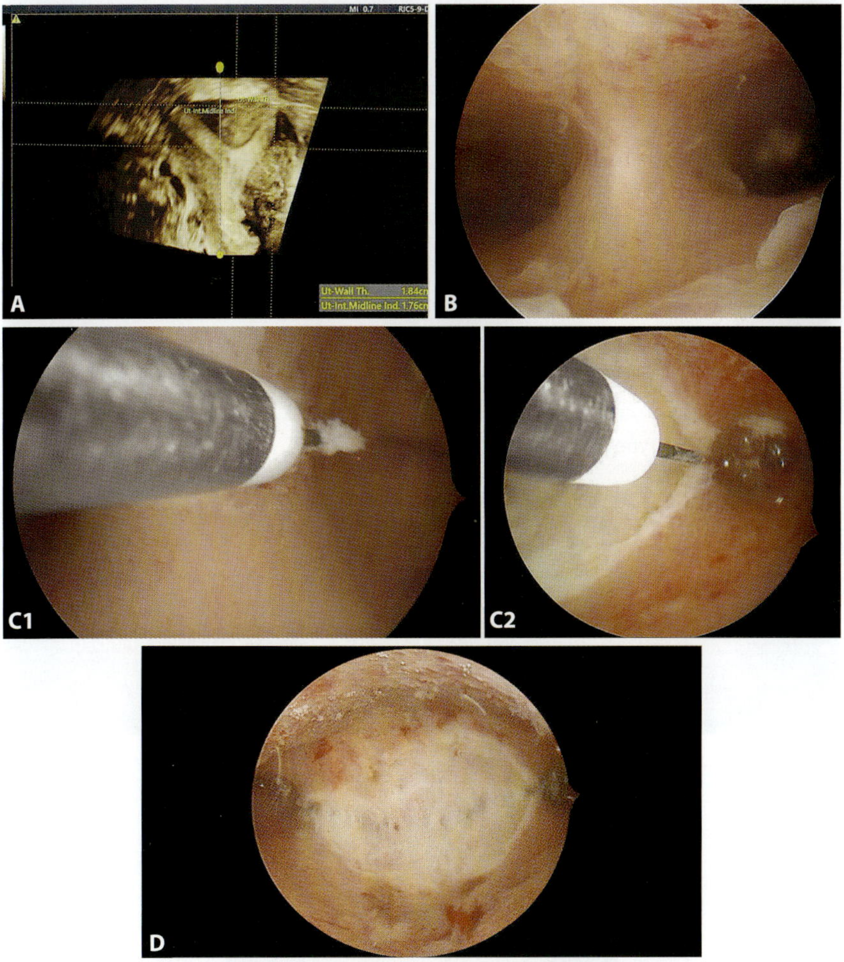

Figs. 7A to D: Septum. (A) Partial septum; (B) Hysteroscopic view of partial septum; (C: 1-2) Hysteroscopic excision of partial septum using bipolar electrode needle. Incision is taken in the midline keeping the ostia as the reference point septum is excised until both ostia are visualized; and (D) Final view after septum resection.

If Vasovagal occurs: Stop procedure, put the patient in supine position, legs elevated, oxygen and atropine if bradycardia.

CONTRAINDICATIONS

- *Absolute:* Active pelvic infection, Confirmed pregnancy

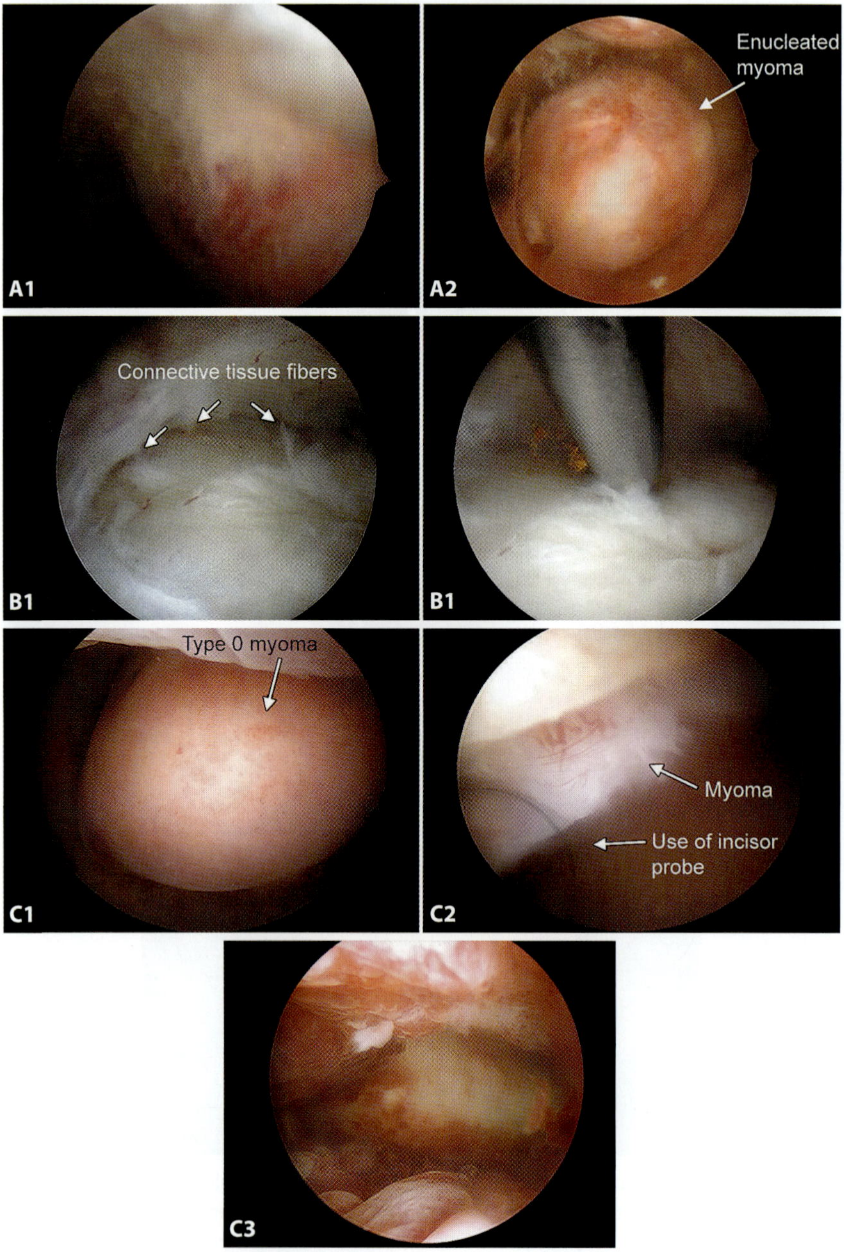

Figs. 8A to C

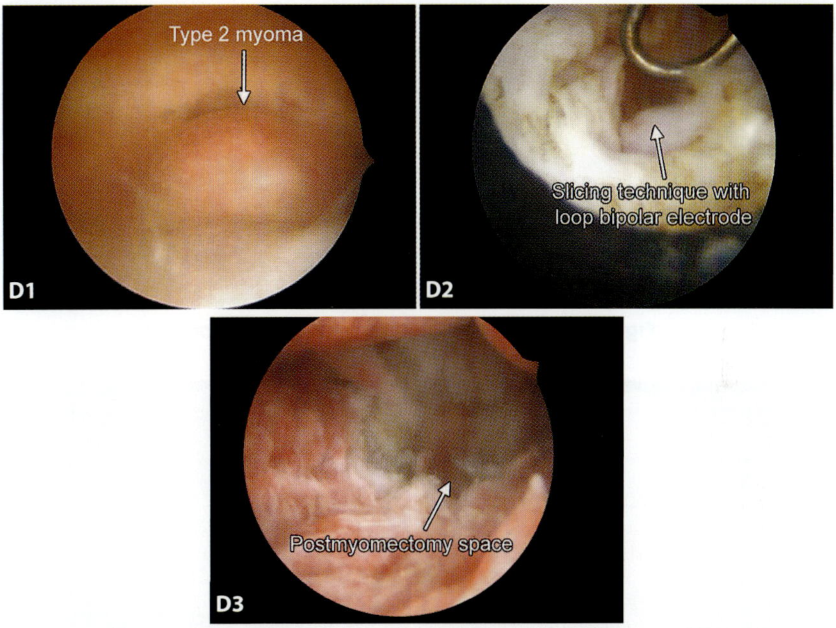

Figs. 8A to D: Submucous fibroids. (A: 1 and 2) Type 1 Anterior wall fibroid; (B: 1-3) Enucleation of the fibroid using scissors; (C: 1-3) In Office Hysteroscopic myomectomy using tissue removal system; (D: 1-3) In office Hysteroscopic myomectomy using 16 Fr resectoscope with loop bipolar electrode.

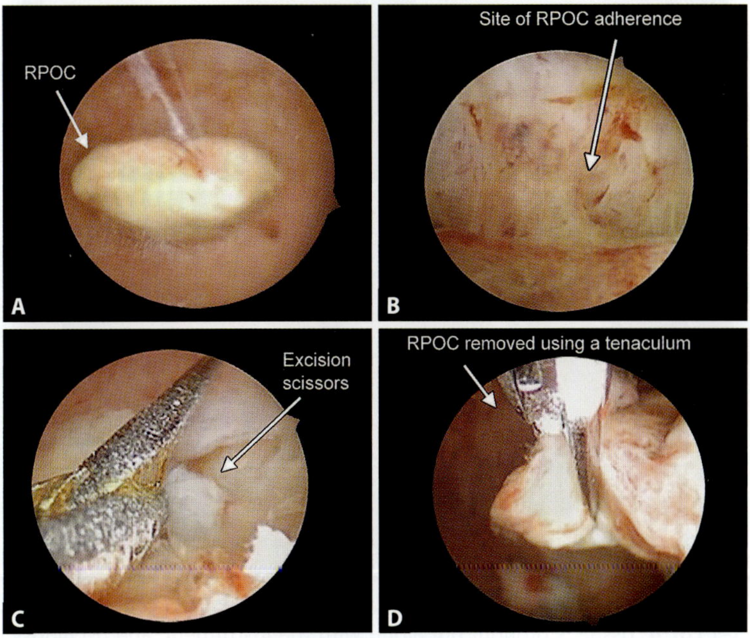

Figs. 9A to D

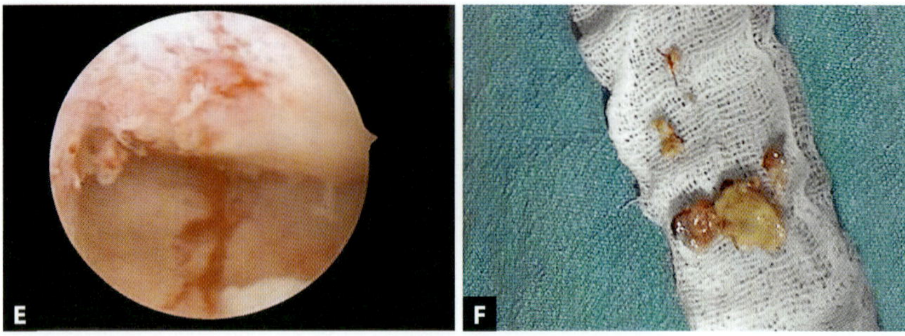

Figs. 9A to F: RPOC—RPOC removal with scissors.

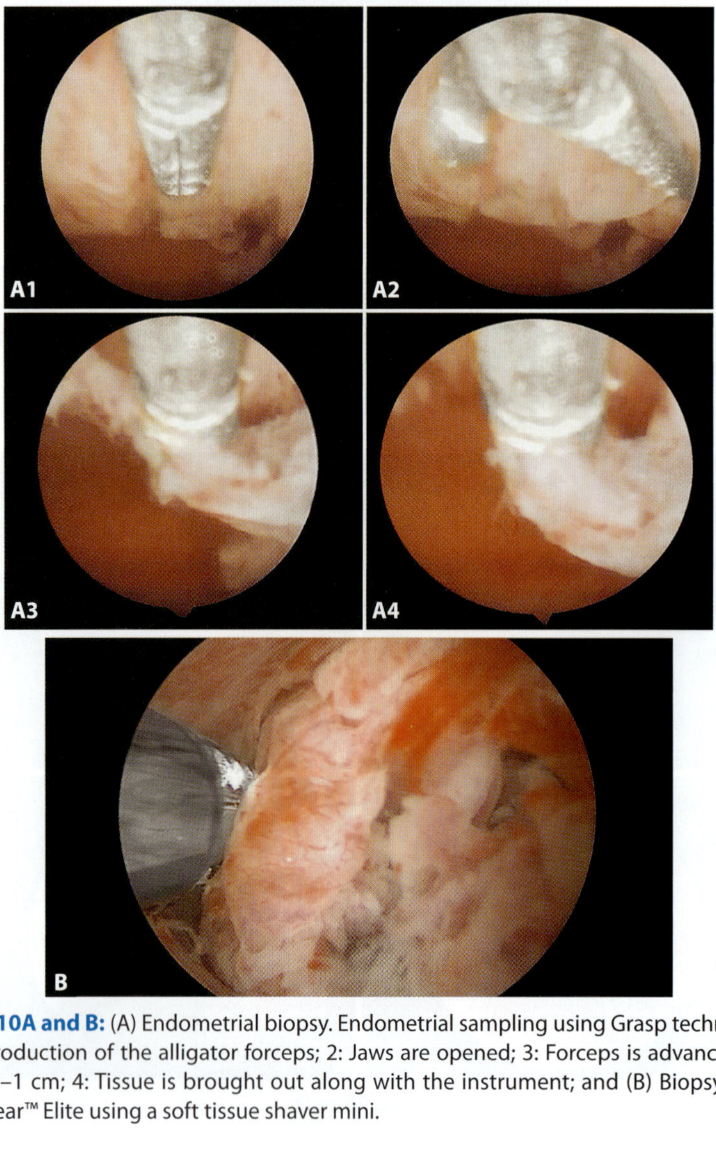

Figs. 10A and B: (A) Endometrial biopsy. Endometrial sampling using Grasp technique. 1: Introduction of the alligator forceps; 2: Jaws are opened; 3: Forceps is advanced up to 0.5–1 cm; 4: Tissue is brought out along with the instrument; and (B) Biopsy with TruClear™ Elite using a soft tissue shaver mini.

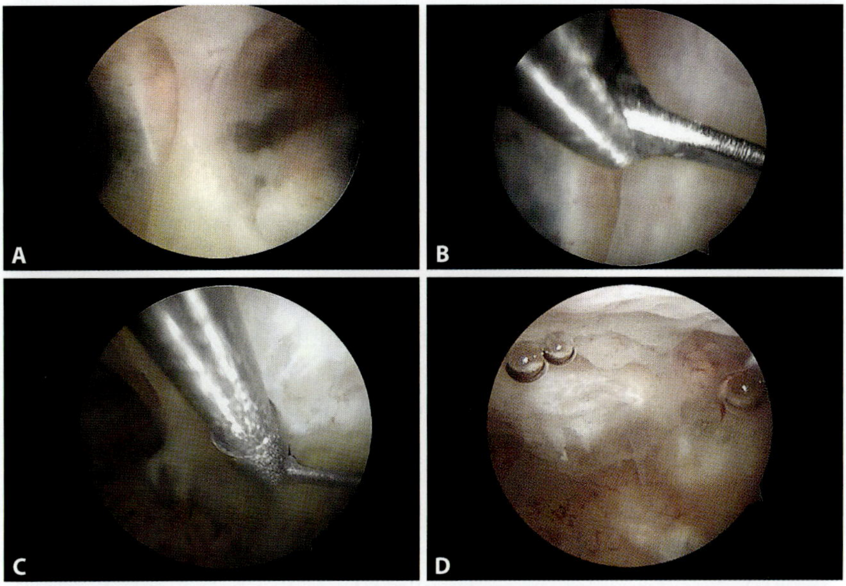

Figs. 11A to D: Intrauterine adhesions—Adhesiolysis done using 5 Fr scissors.

TABLE 5: In office hysteroscopy.

Innovation	*Impact*
Miniaturized hysteroscopes (≤2 mm)	Improved patient tolerance
Bipolar energy	Saline as distension medium; safer
Morcellation systems (Truclear®. Bigatti shaver)	Faster tissue removal
3D/4K visualization	Enhanced diagnostic precision
AI and Virtual Reality (VR)	Patient education and anxiety reduction

- *Relative:* Heavy active bleeding (may obscure view), Severe cervical stenosis

Post-procedure Care

- Observe for 15–30 minutes for delayed vasovagal symptoms
- Advise light activity for 24 hours
- Inform about mild spotting or cramping
- Report excessive bleeding, fever, or pain

***Table 5** will explain about the innovations and impact in office hysteroscopy.*

VIRTUAL REALITY IN OFFICE HYSTEROSCOPY

Preoperative VR education has shown to *reduce anxiety and pain perception* by improving patient preparedness.

In a pilot study (Tanvir et al., 2024), VR-based pre-procedural videos were associated with a significant reduction in preoperative anxiety scores ($p < 0.05$).

TABLE 6: Key messages.

Do's	*Don'ts*
Use small-diameter scopes	Avoid routine cervical dilation
Ensure patient comfort and privacy	Do not rush the entry
Continuous flow and steady pressure	Avoid blind biopsy
Record procedure for audit/training	Don't ignore patient distress cues
Maintain low intrauterine pressure	Avoid routine anesthesia

Mechanism: VR → Familiarization with procedure → Reduced anticipatory anxiety → Decreased sympathetic activation

Table 6 will explain about do's and don'ts while performing hysteroscopy.

CONCLUSION

Office hysteroscopy is a cornerstone of modern gynecology. With proper technique, equipment, and patient communication, young gynecologists can safely integrate it into everyday clinical practice to improve diagnostic accuracy and patient satisfaction.

SUGGESTED READING

1. Bettocchi S, Di Spiezio Sardo A, Ceci O, et al. Hysteroscopy without anesthesia: review of 4863 cases. J Am Assoc Gynecol Laparosc. 2002;9(3): 283-6.
2. Bettocchi S, Nappi L, Ceci O, Selvaggi L. Office hysteroscopy. Obstet Gynecol Clin North Am. 2004;31(1):641-54.
3. Campo R, Van Belle Y, Rombauts Y, Brosens I, Gordts S. Office mini-hysteroscopy. Hum Reprod Update. 1999;5(1):73-81.
4. Clark TJ, Voit D, Gupta JK, Hyde C, Song F, Khan KS. Accuracy of outpatient hysteroscopy in endometrial cancer. BMJ. 2002;325(7376):669.
5. Cooper NA, et al. Pain relief in outpatient hysteroscopy (PRODIGY): a multicenter RCT. BJOG. 2015;122(4):535-41.
6. Di Spiezio Sardo A, Calagna G, et al. The role of modern hysteroscopy in improving patient experience and safety. Best Pract Res Clin Obstet Gynaecol. 2021;77:55-67.
7. Jansen FW, Vredevoogd CB, van Ulzen K, Hermans J, Trimbos JB, Trimbos-Kemper TC. Complications of hysteroscopy: multicenter study. Obstet Gynecol. 2000;96(2):266-70.
8. Moore JF. Hysteroscopy. In: Stat Pearls [Internet]. Treasure Island (FL): Stat Pearls Publishing; 2025.
9. Nagele F, et al. Diagnostic accuracy of office hysteroscopy versus transvaginal sonography in the diagnosis of uterine abnormalities. Obstet Gynecol. 1996;87(3):387-91.
10. Tanvir T, Garzon S, Alonso Pacheco L, Lopez Yarto, Rios M, Stamenov G, et al. Office hysteroscopic myomectomy without myoma extraction: A multicenter prospective study. Eur J Obstet Gynecol Reprod Biol. 2021;256:358-63.
11. Tanvir T et al. Preoperative VR reduces anxiety in office hysteroscopy: pilot study,2025 (unpublished data)

23 CHAPTER

Rare Presentations and Innovations in Hysteroscopy

Sonia Naik

Rare presentations do surprise us but also pose a challenge in the management of the condition. And these challenging situations make interesting case reports.

CASE 1

A 36 years woman with secondary infertility had a workup for infertility. She was Para 1 and had history of one miscarriage in the first trimester. She earlier had a history of rescue cerclage done in her second pregnancy at 17 weeks. She narrates her second pregnancy to be bound to bed after her rescue cerclage. She had been cohabiting with her husband for 4 years and not able to conceive.

She underwent investigations for infertility including hormonal and biochemical profile which were all normal. Her Pap smear was normal. Her husband's semen analysis was good.

Her 3D transvaginal sonography for evaluation of the cavity showed linear hyperechogenicity.

She was planned for hysteroscopy. Hysteroscopy done vaginoscopically showed a bunch of blue threads seen coming into the cervical canal. Further going ahead it showed some threads seen in the lower part of uterine cavity. The ostia were well visualized. The endometrium looking more vascular with fine vessels branching throughout the endometrial cavity. The bluish threads were in a bunch of three to four, they were traced to coming out through myometrium in the lower part of the cavity.

This was further clarified with the patient's family and they then informed that the patient had undergone cerclage which was in emergency and when cervix was 2 cm open. The puzzle was then resolved that these sutures were prolene. Two strands of doubled up prolene was probably used. which was doubled up and used.

The prolene in the lower part of the uterine cavity and that coming out into the cervical canal actually behaved as a foreign body and was the reason for infertility.

CASE 2

A Para 1 previous LSCS had secondary infertility for 2 years. She had a Mirena insertion after the first childbirth which was 7 years back. She got the Mirena removed 2 years back and blamed Mirena for not been able to get pregnant. Periods remained scanty after removal of Mirena. The Mirena was also blamed to be the cause of scanty periods. Hormonal profile was done to rule out any hormonal abnormality.

Hysteroscopy was done as a part of workup for secondary infertility and also scanty periods. Vaginoscopic hysteroscopy revealed tight internal os negotiated with difficulty. There were adhesions in the cervical canal which were managed with aquadissection. The uterine cavity was small. The endometrium was thin. There were adhesions covering the right cornua. The adhesions were cut with the scissors. Beyond the adhesions was a white longitudinal 1 cm plastic thing seen embedded in the myometrium. It was then realized that it was a broken horizontal tip of the Mirena. This tip had caused adhesions and therefore the endometrium got thinned out. Therefore the patient had scanty periods. The adhesions were cut and the cavity reformed. With the help of graspers the Mirena was moved back and forth to dislodge. It was with much efforts that it was dislodged.

The patient was then put on high doses of estrogen for 5 weeks followed by withdrawal. She has started having proper flow. Her tubal patency will be checked henceforth.

Hysteroscopy is the basic tool for infertility workup and a vaginoscopic approach should be a part of curriculum development for all the Postgraduate students.

KEY POINTS

- *Foreign Body-Induced Infertility:* In Case 1, retained prolene sutures from a prior emergency cerclage were identified via hysteroscopy as intrauterine foreign bodies, contributing to secondary infertility.
- *Mirena Fragment Complication:* Case 2 revealed a retained broken horizontal arm of a previously removed Mirena IUD embedded in the myometrium, causing intrauterine adhesions and endometrial thinning, leading to hypomenorrhea and infertility.
- *Diagnostic Value of Hysteroscopy:* Both cases underscore the critical role of vaginoscopic hysteroscopy in identifying subtle or unexpected intrauterine pathology not evident on imaging or routine workup.
- *Therapeutic Intervention:* Adhesiolysis and foreign body removal were successfully performed hysteroscopically in both cases, followed by hormonal therapy to restore endometrial function in Case 2.
- *Training Implication:* These cases highlight the importance of incorporating vaginoscopic hysteroscopy techniques into postgraduate Gynecology training for effective diagnosis and management of complex infertility cases.

SUGGESTING READING

1. ACOG Practice Bulletin No. 142: Cerclage for the Management of Cervical Insufficiency. HYPERLINK "https://www.acog.org/clinical/clinical-guidance/practice-bulletin/articles/2014/02/cerclage-for-the-management-of-cervical-insufficiency"ACOG Practice Bulletin No. 142
2. ASRM Guideline: Evidence-Based Treatments for Unexplained Infertility (2020) Hysteroscopy in the evaluation of unexplained infertility, especially when intrauterine pathology is suspected. HYPERLINK "https://www.asrm.org/practice-guidance/practice-committee-documents/evidence-based-treatments-for-couples-with-unexplained-infertility-a-guideline-2020/"ASRM Unexplained Infertility Guideline.
3. Hysteroscopic Management of Retained Intrauterine Foreign Bodies Journal: Fertility and Sterility PMID: 29551317.
4. Intrauterine Device Fragment Retention: A Rare Cause of Infertility Journal: Case Reports in Obstetrics and Gynecology PMID: 31263489.
5. RCOG Green-top Guideline No. 75: Cervical Cerclage: Reviews evidence for prophylactic and emergency cerclage, including complications such as suture retention and infection. Link: HYPERLINK "https://www.rcog.org.uk/guidance/browse-all-guidance/green-top-guidelines/cervical-cerclage-green-top-guideline-no-75/"RCOG Green-top 75
6. Retained Cerclage Suture Causing Infertility: A Rare Case Report Journal: Journal of Human Reproductive Sciences PMID: 32792712.

24 CHAPTER

Complications of Hysteroscopy

Kalyan B Barmade, Vijay Nahata, Maithili Kumari, Ritu Jain, Aastha Aggarwal

COMPLICATIONS OF HYSTEROSCOPY

Hysteroscopy is a valuable minimally invasive tool for evaluation and management of intrauterine pathology. Despite its safety, several intraoperative and postoperative complications may arise. Early identification, prevention, and prompt management reduce morbidity and improve outcomes. Diagnostic procedures have lower complications than the operative procedures (0.13% vs 0.95%). Overall complication rate for operative hysteroscopy is 2% (AAGL 1993). The greatest risk of complications occurs with Adhesiolysis (4.48%), followed by endometrial resection (0.81%), myomectomy (0.75%), and polypectomy (0.38%).

RISK FACTORS

- *Parity:* Nulliparous women have narrower cervical canals ⇒ ↑ risk of trauma and false passage (RCOG, 2018).
- Extremes of age→ cervical stenosis (Munro et al., 2014).
- *Previous cervical surgery:* LEEP, cone biopsy → fibrosis and stenosis; risk of false track formation.
- *Uterine position:* Extreme anteversion or retroversion can distort cervical-uterine axis (Campo et al., 2011).
- Severe Intrauterine Adhesions
- *Fibroids:* Cervical or isthmic fibroids can alter the canal pathway.
- Inadequate experience with vaginoscopic entry
- Forceful insertion of dilators or hysteroscope
- Poor alignment of cervical-uterine axis

IMMEDIATE COMPLICATIONS

- *Failure to enter:* Occurs due to either cervical stenosis, abnormal uterine position, or obscured view. Office hysteroscopy accounts for 4.2% of all failures. Procedure can be abandoned if done as an outpatient procedure, or cervical ripening should be done preoperatively, or use of USG guidance **(Flowchart 1)**.

Flowchart 1: Trouble shooting in difficult hysteroscopic entry.

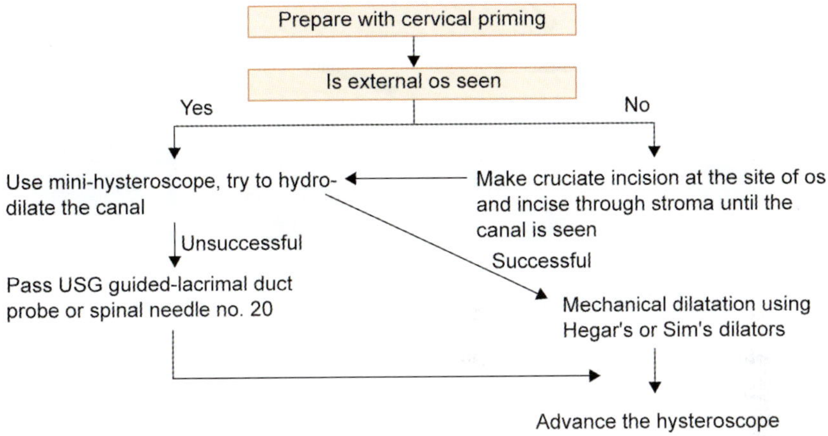

Management:

- *Acutely Ante flexed uterus*; Place a long-bladed speculum deep in the anterior or posterior fornix, it pushes the fundus to the mid position and can facilitate dilation.
- *Acutely Retroflexed uterus:* Place a vulsellum on the posterior lip of the cervix and apply traction, it straightens the cervical canal
- *Cervical stenosis:* Preoperative cervical priming with agents:
  - Misoprostol 400 mg either orally or vaginally 6-8 hours prior to surgery or 400 mg sublingually 2–4 hours prior to surgery.
  - *Hygroscopic dilators:* Laminaria tents 12 hours before procedure
  - Intracervical injection of vasopressin solution (4 IU in 100 cc sodium chloride) injected at the 4 and 8 o'clock positions.

- *Cervical trauma/Laceration:* Occurs when significant traction is used on handling surgical instruments applied to the cervix (holding with tenaculum or vulsellum), or in cervical stenosis patients. Pressure with a swab or stick, in some cases cervical suturing may be required. Preoperative cervical ripening agents should be given to avoid Recommendation is to perform Vaginoscopy by "no touch technique" (Bettocchi et al., 2004), Gentle, slow advancement, use of smaller diameter scopes (<5 mm)
- *False Passage:* Occurs when the hysteroscope deviates from the cervical canal, creating a false tract. Risk factors include cervical stenosis and improper alignment. Prevention involves gentle dilation, use of a tenaculum, and avoiding forceful entry **(Fig. 1)**.
- *Perforation:* Defined as accidental penetration of the uterine wall by hysteroscope or instruments. incidence is 14 per 1,000 (AAGL survey) Perforation is more common in repeat procedures like Adhesiolysis.

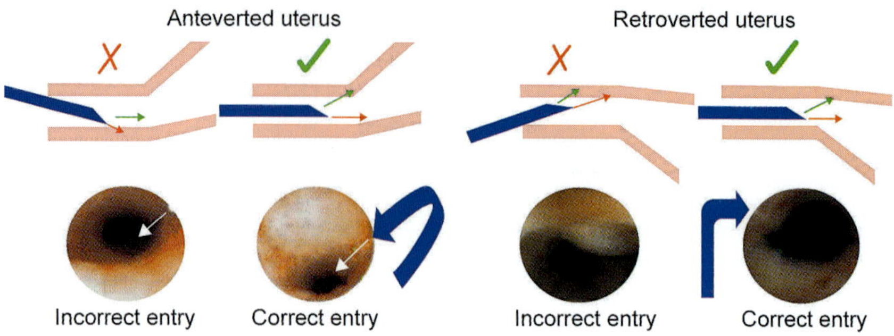

Fig. 1: Hysteroscopic entry in anteverted and retroverted uterus.

Flowchart 2: Management in various types of hysteroscopic perforation.

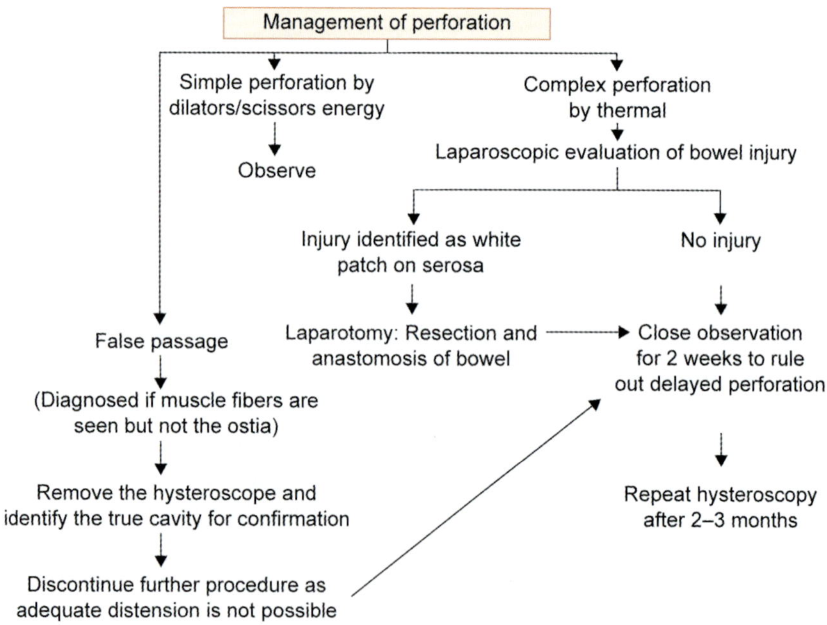

Risk factors include postmenopausal uterus, scarring, or excessive force, Misalignment of cervical and uterine axis, Insertion against resistance, Adhesiolysis (Asherman's syndrome). Suspect if loss of resistance or sudden loss of visualization occurs. Management involves stopping the procedure, assessing with laparoscopy, and monitoring for visceral injury **(Flowchart 2)**.

Tips to avoid creating a false passage or perforation:

- Vaginoscopy should be performed
- Dilate the cervix with slow, steady pressure and stop when internal os opens, dilators should not be pushed to fundus

  - Hydrostatic dilatation with inflow "on" and outflow "off" must be preferred.
  - Always insert the hysteroscope or resectoscope under direct vision.
- *Bleeding:* Usually results from cervical trauma or intrauterine injury or laceration of cervical branch/arcuate/uterine artery. Minor bleeding may resolve with pressure or coagulation, while severe bleeding may require tamponade or surgical repair. Applying a hysteroscope tip or placing a foley balloon (10–30 mi) works as effective tamponade.
- *Vision Difficulty:* Caused by bleeding, inadequate distension, or fogging. Ensure clear fluid inflow and outflow and maintain visualization throughout the procedure.
- *Difficulty in Distension:* Occurs due to leakage, obstruction, or uterine perforation. Check tubing, verify correct intrauterine placement, and adjust pressure appropriately.
- *Retrieval Issues:* Failure to retrieve tissue or device fragments may occur. Always perform under-vision removal and confirm clearance hysteroscopically.
- *Breakage of Instruments:* Breakage may occur from excessive force or defective instruments. Prevention includes pre-use inspection and proper maintenance. Retrieve fragments under direct vision.
- *Fluid overload* during hysteroscopy, known as operative hysteroscopy intravascular absorption (OHIA) syndrome, can lead to serious, potentially fatal, complications such as *pulmonary edema, cerebral edema, heart failure, and severe electrolyte imbalances.*

Complications of Fluid Overload: The complications depend on the type of distending media used (hypotonic vs. isotonic).

- *With Hypotonic Solutions (e.g., 1.5% Glycine, 3% Sorbitol):* Excessive absorption of these electrolyte-free fluids causes water to move into cells due to an osmotic gradient.
  - *Hyponatremia and Hypo-osmolality:* Dilution of serum sodium and other electrolytes.
  - *Cerebral Edema:* Swelling of brain cells can cause nausea, vomiting, headache, visual disturbances, confusion, seizures, coma, permanent brain damage, or death.
  - *Cardiovascular Issues:* Pulmonary edema, heart failure, bradycardia, and hypotension.
- *With Isotonic Solutions (e.g., 0.9% Normal Saline):* Although less likely to cause electrolyte imbalance, excessive absorption can still lead to volume overload.
  - *Volume Overload:* Can cause pulmonary edema, laryngeal edema, congestive heart failure, and hypertension.

- *Metabolic Acidosis:* Large volumes of normal saline can cause hyperchloremic metabolic acidosis.

Prevention of Fluid Overload: Prevention focuses on minimizing fluid absorption and diligent monitoring.

- *Monitor Fluid Balance:* A designated individual must meticulously track the difference between infused and outflowing fluid volumes (fluid deficit) at least every 10 minutes.
- *Use Appropriate Media:* The ACOG recommends using isotonic solutions like normal saline with bipolar electrosurgery to reduce the risk of hyponatremia.
- *Limit Intrauterine Pressure:* Maintain the lowest possible intrauterine pressure necessary for visualization (ideally below 70 mm Hg).
- *Implement Fluid Deficit Thresholds:* Stop the procedure if the fluid deficit reaches specific limits:
  - *Healthy patients:* 1,000 mL for hypotonic solutions, 2,500 mL for isotonic solutions.
  - *High-risk patients (elderly, cardiac, or renal comorbidities):* 750 mL for hypotonic solutions, 1,500 mL for isotonic solutions.
- *Minimize Procedure Duration:* Prolonged operative times (ideally under 1 hour) increase the risk of absorption.
- *Consider adjunctive measures:*
  - *Regional Anesthesia:* Allows early detection of symptoms like restlessness or headache, which may be masked by general anesthesia.
  - *Vasopressin Injection:* Intracervical injection of dilute vasopressin can help reduce fluid absorption.

Management of Fluid Overload: Prompt action is crucial if fluid overload is suspected.

- *Terminate the Procedure:* Stop the surgery, cease fluid infusion, and deflate the uterus.
- *Assess and Monitor:* Immediately evaluate the patient's hemodynamic, neurological, and respiratory status. Insert a Foley catheter to monitor urine output and order immediate blood tests for serum electrolytes (especially sodium), osmolality, and renal function.
- *Provide supportive care:*
  - Administer supplemental oxygen; intubation and mechanical ventilation may be necessary for respiratory distress or pulmonary edema.
  - Manage blood pressure; vasopressors may be needed for hypotension.

- *Administer Diuretics:* Intravenous loop diuretics, such as furosemide, are typically administered to treat volume overload and pulmonary edema.
- *Correct Electrolyte Imbalance:* For severe or symptomatic hyponatremia, a controlled infusion of 3% hypertonic saline may be required under specialist guidance to slowly correct sodium levels and avoid complications like osmotic demyelination syndrome.

Effective communication and teamwork among the surgical and anesthesia teams are essential for early recognition and management of this life-threatening condition.

LATE COMPLICATIONS

- *Endometritis:* Postoperative infection leading to fever, pelvic pain, and discharge. Managed with broad-spectrum antibiotics and adequate drainage if needed.
- *Hematometra:* Blood accumulation within the uterine cavity secondary to obstruction or adhesions. Presents with cyclic pain and amenorrhea. Managed with cervical dilation or adhesiolysis
- *Intrauterine Synechiae (Asherman's Syndrome):* Adhesions within the uterine cavity due to trauma or infection. May cause infertility, amenorrhea, or oligomenorrhea. Managed with hysteroscopic adhesiolysis.
- *Placenta Accreta Spectrum (PAS):* Scarring following hysteroscopic surgery may predispose to abnormal placentation in future pregnancies. Requires antenatal vigilance and multidisciplinary management.

Flowchart 3: Prevention and management of hysteroscopic complications.

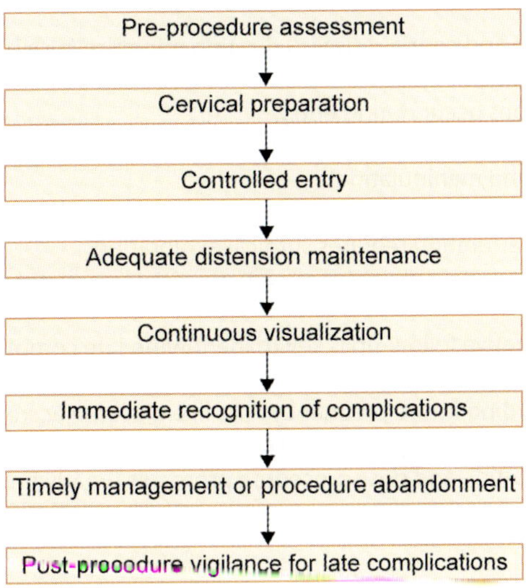

TABLE 1: Major complications and their management.

Complication	*Management approach*
False Passage	Stop procedure, reattempt under guidance, reassess anatomy and enter with smaller scope, avoid forceful entry
Perforation	Stop procedure, evaluate extent, monitor or repair if indicated
Bleeding	Pressure, coagulation, tamponade, or surgical intervention
Breakage of Instruments	Inspect and maintain instruments Retrieved under vision
Vision Difficulty	Ensure proper distension; control bleeding, clean optics, Irrigation
Difficulty in Distension	Check tubing, ensure intrauterine placement, adjust pressure; rule out perforation; close cervix with tenaculum
Retrieval Issues	Remove under vision and confirm complete clearance, use suction evacuation if necessary
Late Complications	Antibiotics for infection; Adhesiolysis for synechiae; careful follow-up in subsequent pregnancies

(**Flowchart 3**: Prevention and Management of Hysteroscopic Complications)

(**Table 1**: Overview of Major Hysteroscopic Complications and Its Management)

KEY POINTS

- Hysteroscopy, though safe, carries a risk of both immediate and delayed complications.
- Proper technique and continuous visualization minimize false passage, perforation, and bleeding.
- Most complications occur during entry.
- Proper cervical preparation reduces trauma.
- Avoid forceful blind manipulation.
- Ultrasound aids safe entry in difficult cases.
- Electrosurgical perforation requires surgical exploration.
- Instrument care and flow maintenance are essential to prevent mechanical and visual problems.
- Vigilant postoperative follow-up is key to identifying late complications such as infection, synechiae, and hematometra.
- Counseling regarding future pregnancy risks like placenta accreta spectrum should be provided to all surgical candidates.
- Structured pre-, intra-, and post-procedure protocols greatly improve patient safety and outcomes.

SUGGESTED READING

1. ACOG. The Use of Hysteroscopy for the Diagnosis and Treatment of Intrauterine Pathology. ACOG Committee Opinion. Number 800. Obstet Gynecol. 2020; 135(3):e138-48.
2. American Association of Gynecologic Laparoscopists. AAGL Practice Report: Practice Guidelines for the Diagnosis and Management of Endometrial Polyps. J Minim Invasive Gynecol. 2020;27(2):237-53.
3. Bettocchi S, Selvaggi L. Hysteroscopy: An operative approach to intrauterine pathology. Baillieres Clin Obstet Gynaecol. 2000;14(4):845-57.
4. Bradley LD. Cutting the risk of hysteroscopic complications. OBG Manag. 2004;16(1):44-52.
5. Campo R, et al. Hysteroscopy: Current status and future directions. Hum Reprod Update. 2018;24(5):557-74.
6. Di Spiezio Sardo A, et al. Hysteroscopic surgery: safety considerations and new perspectives. Facts Views Vis Obgyn. 2019;11(3):211-9.
7. Elahmedawy H, Snook NJ. Complications of operative hysteroscopy: an anaesthetist's perspective. BJA Educ. 2021;21(7):240-2.
8. Emanuel MH. Complications of hysteroscopic surgery. Best Pract Res Clin Obstet Gynaecol. 2013;27(6):743-53.
9. ESGE Guideline on Hysteroscopy. Facts Views Vis ObGyn.
10. Glasser MH. Hysteroscopy: Managing and minimizing operative complications. OBG Manag. 2005;17(2):42-57.
11. Hoffman CR, Van Hal M, Tariq R, George S. Complications of fluid overload during hysteroscopic surgery. Korean J Anesthesiol. 2019;72(4):387-8.
12. Hooker AB, et al. Long-term complications, and reproductive outcome after hysteroscopic surgery. Hum Reprod Update. 2018;24(6):702-17.
13. Jansen FW, Vredevoogd CB, van Ulzen K, Hermans J, Trimbos JB, Trimbos-Kemper TC. Complications of hysteroscopy: a prospective, multicenter study. Obstet Gynecol. 2000;96(2):266-70.
14. Jauniaux E, Collins S, Burton GJ. Placenta accreta spectrum disorders after uterine surgery. Am J Obstet Gynecol. 2019;221(6):483-99.
15. Lasmar RB. Hysteroscopic complications: causes and prevention. J Minim Invasive Gynecol. 2020;27(6):1206-15.
16. Lee EB, Park J, Lim HK, Kim YI, Jin Y, Lee KH. Complications of fluid overload during hysteroscopic surgery: cardiomyopathy and epistaxis - A case report. Anesth Pain Med (Seoul). 2020;15(1):61-5.
17. Manchanda R, Sharma R. Hysteroscopy simplified by masters. Chapter Complications of Hysteroscopy and Management. Berlin; Springer Nature; 2020. pp. 211-22.
18. Mazzon I, Favilli A. Complications in hysteroscopic surgery: prevention and management. Best Pract Res Clin Obstet Gynaecol. 2021;75:40-53.
19. RCOG Green-top Guideline on Hysteroscopy.
20. Yu D, Wong YM, Cheong Y, Xia E, Li TC. Asherman syndrome — one century later. Fertil Steril. 2008;89(4):759-79.